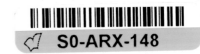

SIMPLE STRENGTH

Mercedes Pollmeier

Digital Photography by Aaron Rourke
Videography by Truc Allen
Edited by Kate Strickland and Laura Praderio
Mercedes Pollmeier Headshot by Nathan Hadley

Book Layout © 2015 MyAuthorlyFormatting.com
Cover Design by Ida Fia Sveningsson

ISBN 978-1515176237

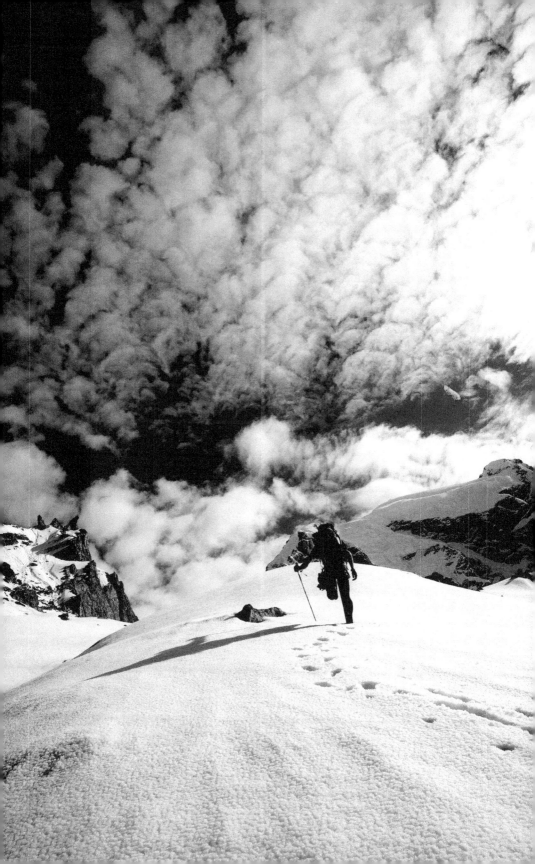

Master these movements to become the best athlete you can be. Use the accompanying programs to get the most out of this book. Get them for free at www.SimpleStrengthBook.com.

Work hard and stay strong

—Mercedes Pollmeier

Dedicated to My Loving and Supportive Wife

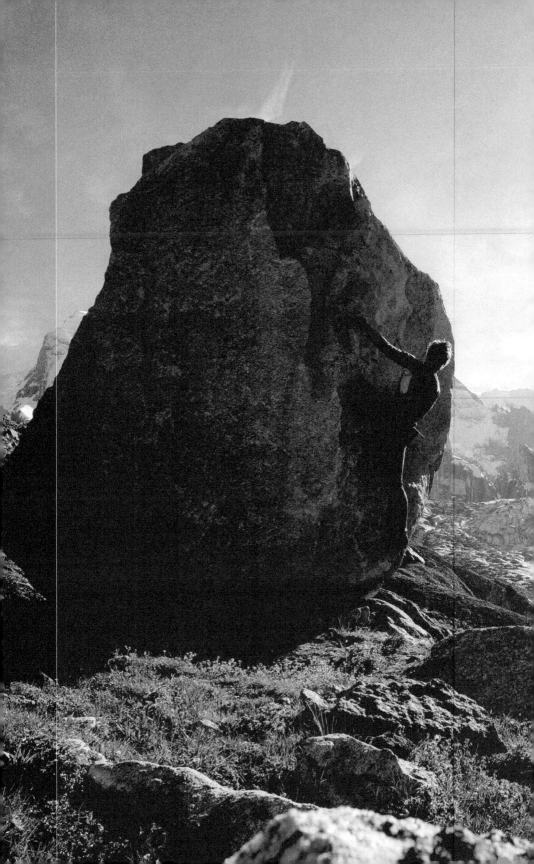

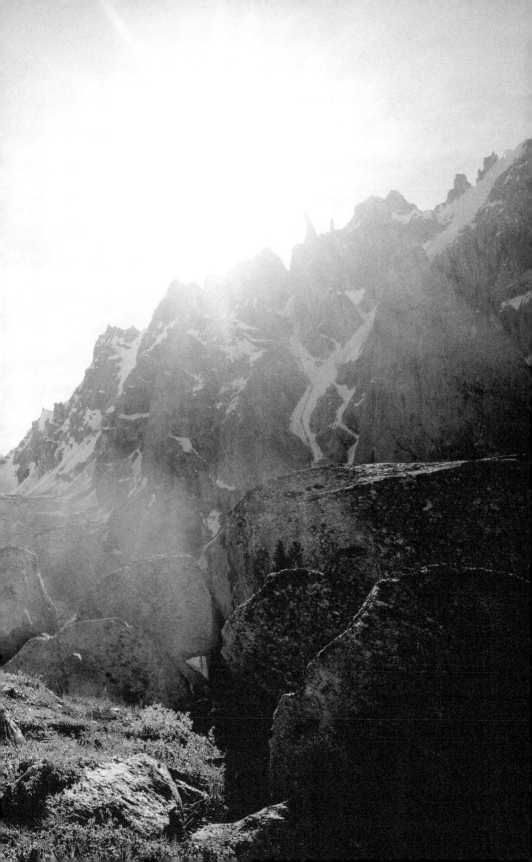

DISCLAIMER

All the information presented in *Simple Strength* is for educational and resource purposes *only*. It is *not* a substitute for or an addition to any advice given to you by your Physician or Health Care Provider.

Before making any changes to your lifestyle, diet, and exercise habits and before implementing any information in *Simple Strength*, you must consult your Physician. Please understand that *you* are solely responsible for the way information in the Simple Strength book is perceived and utilized and you do so at your own risk.

In no way will *Simple Strength/Mercedes Pollmeier* or any persons associated with Simple Strength be held responsible for any injuries and problems that may occur due to the use of this book or the advice contained within. *Simple Strength/Mercedes Pollmeier* will not be held responsible for the conduct of any companies and websites recommended within this book.

CONTENTS

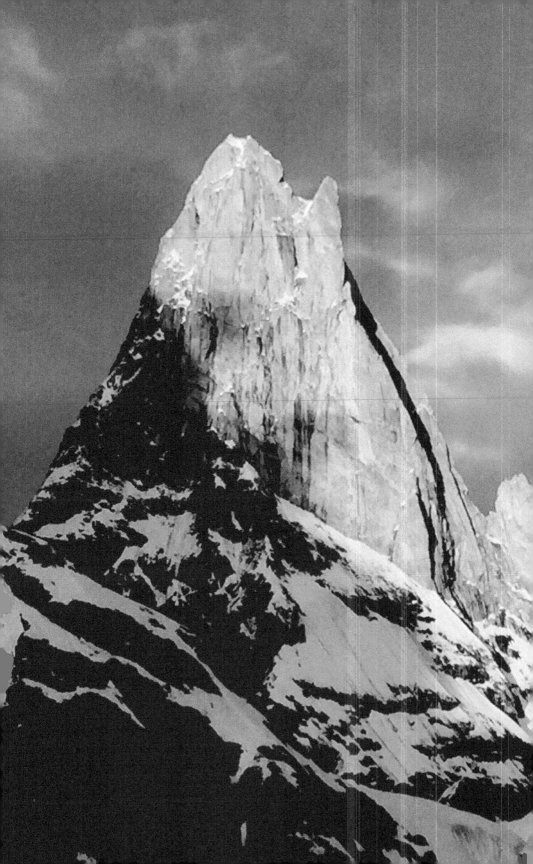

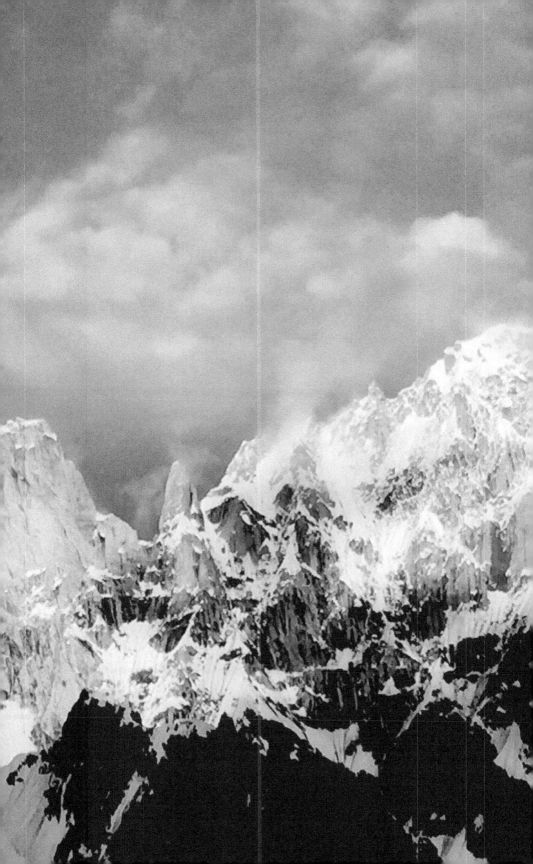

SECTION ONE

FOREWORD BY GRAHAM ZIMMERMAN

As an alpine climbing athlete, training for expeditions is a very important part of what I do. When I am home in Bend, Oregon, I train in a facility utilizing a wide range of equipment, but due to my lifestyle and line of work I am more often than not in a location where I don't have access to the resources that make following a routine easy. And so the question presented itself: How do I gain and maintain the strength needed to climb hard routes while training with minimal equipment?

In 2013, I posed this to Mercedes and we worked together to build a training routine that would allow me to train while on the road like I was at my home gym. Once familiar with my new regimen, I was able to travel with only a hang board and yoga mat while still making significant strength gains, particularly in my core and stabilizing muscles.

A year later, I traveled to the Alaska Range after a long stint of training on the road. During the trip, my partner and I intended to make the first ascent of the West face of Titanic peak in the Revelations sub range. With 4,000 feet of relief, this face would generally be considered a candidate for a multi-day climb, but with the fitness gained from the training regimen developed by Mercedes, we were able to complete the route in a 22.5-hour push from camp. As one might imagine, we were psyched.

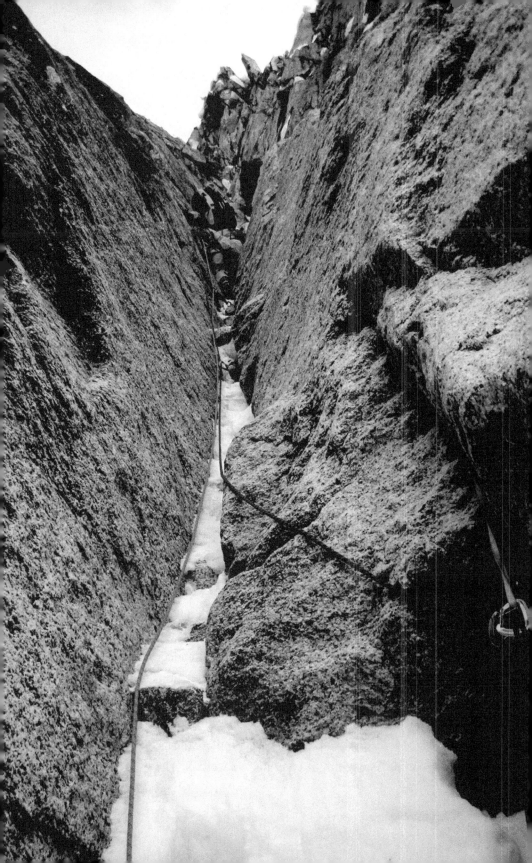

At the end of my spring season in Alaska I took a fall that resulted in a torn ACL in my right knee. During the ensuing 10 months of physical therapy I was able to utilize many of the elements of the bodyweight training program designed by Mercedes to assist with my recovery. Utilizing these techniques in combination with my prescribed PT, I was able to regain strength quickly and effectively. I am happy to report that I am currently 11 months post surgery and stronger than I have ever been, ready to meet more of my climbing goals in the greater ranges.

"For the last several years, my mountaineering training has consisted of traditional weight lifting, cardio work and hiking. But when I started rock climbing outside and in the gym I was pretty limited because I wasn't able to move the way I needed. The bodyweight exercises that Mercedes customized for me helped me engage and strengthen muscles that I was underutilizing. The program has dramatically helped with my stability, balance, endurance and overall movement in only a short amount of time. Incorporating these into my training routine has made me a stronger and more durable climber." - Jeff Marcell

INTRODUCTION

Does a busy schedule make it next to impossible to get to a gym for cross training as an outdoor athlete? Do you find it challenging to come up with an exercise routine that you know will get you stronger for your lifestyle or sport? Do you feel like your body is "stuck," but increased mobility could help you perform better? If you answered yes to any of these questions, then Simple Strength can show you how to resolve these issues. In this book, I will show you the best exercises for outdoor athletes that require no equipment, less time and focus on the best technique so that your strength gains will come faster and you will move more intentionally and efficiently.

As an outdoor athlete, it is imperative to round out your training with strength and mobility work, but commuting to a gym can be a burden. Sometimes, with a busy schedule you just don't have extra time to commit to going to the gym for an hour of strength training. Or, when you do have time, you may not have the right technique or focus, which makes you less efficient in your overall movement.

Imagine:

You drive several hours to your crag, hike up the approach, start to warm up, and then begin climbing. You get to the crux of your route, and then you can't make the move because you are too tired and feel like you have no strength. You probably just said to yourself, "I should have been training for this!" You feel upset that you didn't train and think, "What have I been doing with my time at the gym?" or, "How will I find the time to get to a gym?"

Or:

You ascended a big-ass mountain, hiked, climbed, ran, skied up and down this thing, enjoyed every single minute of the suffering and then the weekend is over. Now, it is time to start the week again, so you get up early to get in your aerobic workout, work long hours, come home to your loved ones who you haven't seen all weekend (or, if you are lucky, you have a partner that goes on adventures with you), spend a little bit of time with them and then it's time for bed and you start it all over again. But you feel guilty because you didn't find time to fit in strength training or mobility work that you know will make you feel better and that will leave you less sore after each weekend.

"Practice makes Permanent" - Kelley Starrett, MobilityWod

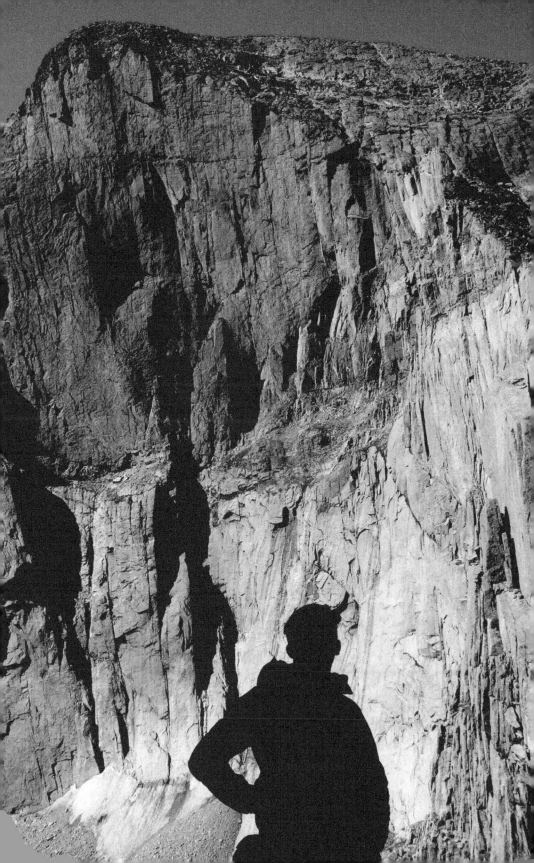

The Cascade

If you practice good movement, you will move better. If you move better, you become more efficient. If you become more efficient, you have greater work capacity, which means you can work harder for longer. If you do harder work for longer, you can push your physical limits. And this all means that you become a beast. For some, this is the goal, and for others, just moving better and being pain free is bliss. So wherever your movement path eventually takes you, by following the steps outlined in this book, I know you will move freer, with more confidence and strength.

> *"Mastering others is strength. Mastering yourself is true power"* - Lao Tzu

Posture and Grace

Have you ever seen a slouchy Olympic sprinter? What about an ungraceful professional dancer? Do you ever see a slouched person move well and gracefully? It should be obvious; good movement and posture are essential for grace and performance, and something that anyone can attain.

From Scrawny to Brawny

> *Peter came to me saying he hadn't done a full squat in decades. He is a backcountry skier, 58 years old and gets by with great skiing technique. The year prior, he did a spring ski trip to Inter Glacier on Mt. Rainier. He hiked up 6,000 feet with skis and then continued to skin up to Steamboat Prow, finishing at 9,700 feet, and then descended in the same fashion. But he felt aches and pains in his knees during the descent, and noticed a lack of stamina on the slopes. What he lacked was mobility and strength in his legs and core. His initial assessment revealed a squat degree of just above 90 degrees; if he went any lower, his back would round and his heels would come up off the ground. We worked on this for a few weeks, and then reassessed. He was able to go all the way down into a full squat, with an assist, without any pain. Peter's stability as well as his knee pain got better over time. He was stronger on his skiing days, lasted longer and was amazed when he went back to repeat Inter Glacier on Mt. Rainier that he had no pain in his knees.*

Peter is just one example of many that have benefited from bodyweight strength and mobility exercises. I also work with a lot of climbers, whose main focus is recruiting the correct pulling muscles (This isn't covered in this book, but you can visit my site, ModusAthletica.com, for more information). For climbers, it's also imperative to not gain any weight during training, but instead to focus on strength and efficiency. Almost all the climbers I work with get stronger and increase their shoulder mobility and are able to climb harder because of this. Hard work pays off.

Making Small Adjustments

As a strength coach, I get to analyze many people's movements. Each person is different, which means every mobility problem will appear differently. However, we can all train to habituate correct movement patterns for our own body. For me, I realized that my standing position for the full squat was a bit too narrow, which prevented me from moving correctly with glutes engaged and proper knee tracking. I took my stance a bit wider and can now move more efficiently through the whole exercise. With small tweaks and adjustments, we can get stronger and move better.

Being Intentional

I've been training and coaching for years, and mostly sport-specific work, but it wasn't until I realized how important intentional movement was, as well as freedom of movement, that I started focusing on mobility and these very basic human movements. I studied with several amazing teachers of movement and progressed through it myself so that I can practice what I preach and teach these fundamentals to others. When I started teaching these movements, my clients were becoming more efficient and content with their bodies. They saw gains quickly and were able to transfer these movements to more functional activities. Their overall performance increased, they became more confident, worked at a higher capacity and had fewer aches and pains.

The Masters

Movement and mobility have been staple diets of some of the best in performance training and exercise science; for example: Pavel Tsatsouline - the master of Russian kettlebell training; Scott Sonnen - the master of mobility work as an MMA fighter; Ido Portal - the master of grace and finesse in parkour and capoeira. What do they all have in common? The ability to use their own bodyweight to increase their skills and strength for overall performance improvement. My goal is to bring many of their ideas together with my own experience and present these exercises in the most efficient way possible for you.

Execute the Fundamentals Well

After you read this, you will see these basic movements as much more than just basic. You will learn that the fundamentals are the most important aspect to master because if you can do these well, you can do most other movements well too. After trying these movements for just a few minutes a day, you will notice a big difference in your hip, spine and shoulder mobility, as well as shoulder, leg and core strength and control. But be warned: you will have to learn these movements with a whole new mind frame, cueing yourself into correct patterns. But I guarantee that if you commit to a new way of thinking about basic movement, it will become easier with time and you will be a better-moving human being.

I will show you how to perform these simple exercises, breaking down each movement so that you can increase your mobility by moving intentionally, and getting stronger by increasing tension throughout the movement. By being intentional about movement and working on the basics, you can become a movement machine, the best version of yourself, and your future self will thank you.

I challenge you to start the movements right away as you read through these pages. You don't have to wait for the right time, or to implement a program. None of these exercises require any equipment, except for your bodyweight and a willingness to learn. Practice small segments each day, and you will gain more mobility and strength, even for the desk-bound athlete. At the end of the book there are programs that you can follow, but honestly, just take 2 minutes per movement each day and work on it. That's only six minutes a day! So what are you waiting for? Let's do this thing!

> *"Don't get stuck in bad positions, guide your body through movements that it is built and made to do. Go there, go all the way there, and that is where the magic happens."* - Mercedes Pollmeier

MY BACKGROUND

I am an athlete who loves my job, and is willing to learn, take risks and face my fears. I constantly crave new information about training, how to build habits, learn new movements and have fun with what I do. Despite education, mentors, injuries and hundreds of clients, I still have so much to learn. I know that I don't know everything about movement, and I hope that day never comes, because that will be the day I lose my passion.

To Understand My Training, You Must Know Where I Came From
I grew up as a competitive tennis player, in Australia, attended an all-girls school that dominated the region, and then eventually landed myself a scholarship in the United States to become a student athlete playing Division I tennis. All I ever wanted was to become a professional tennis player. I thought I either had to become a pro or go to school —the US gave me the opportunity to do both.

The first college I played for was University of Northern Iowa. It was interesting, but I was faced with more challenges than just having to play tennis and get good grades. There was inter-team rivalry that I wouldn't consider healthy. There was racial tension, status issues and "high school" drama. It wasn't what I signed up for, not why I loved tennis. After a year and a half, I started looking for another college to play for. I learned a lot during this time, and it was actually in Iowa where I was first introduced to climbing. At UNI, we had the UNIDome. They had amazing recreational programming, and one of these programs was climbing. I thought that climbing was so different than what I did with tennis that I wanted to learn more. I got a job as a safety-tech and belayed people. It was awesome! I also went on climbing trips, slept in tents with dirtbag climbers, and climbed in the rain. This experience was so humbling, exciting and new that I wanted more. I decided to look for colleges in Colorado, where I knew there were more outdoor adventures to be had.

I was lucky. The coaches at Metropolitan State University of Denver were looking for another female for their team and I fit the bill. Not only was the team mostly Australian, I also had an Australian assistant coach. It was meant to be! This was a much better situation, being a part of healthy team dynamic, and being pushed to be better than I was. Eduardo Provencio and Brad Trost were my coaches at the time. They were brilliant and I still hear their words that encouraged us to try hard, take action and do what you love.

I lived in Denver. I played tennis, got good grades while pursuing a degree in Modern Languages and got to climb once every few months at Paradise Rock Gym. I was also coaching tennis at several country clubs around town to make some money. When I graduated, I still wanted to try my hand at the pros, but I was 22 years old with a shoulder injury that I played through and no coach. The Olympics were coming up, and I figured I'd look into what it would take to play for my home country. One thing I realized is that I could play for Mauritius, the country in which I was born. They had a very small tennis team, and most of the players lived in England or France. I called their head coach and asked if I could try out. It was on. I had to find a coach, and get fitter. I remembered that there was a strength and conditioning coach at Paradise Rock gym whose training sessions looked brutal. I knew that this was what I needed to get my butt into gear. This coach's name was Dave Wahl. He was intrigued to be working with me as a tennis player. His background was in motocross and other outdoor and adventure sports. Dave told me that I needed more upper body strength and that I should cross-train with bouldering. I was willing to do anything, although this seemed very intimidating, since all the boulderers looked really, really strong and my arms were scrawny! I would boulder a few hours a week, train with Dave and play tennis to get ready for the tryouts. I went to Mauritius, played a tournament and made it onto the team! It was awesome. The whole tournament was played in the rain, which was some of the worst tennis I had ever played in my life, but it didn't matter, because I still made it.

I came back to the US ready to train for the Olympic tryouts. Only one country can represent the region of the Indian Ocean, so Mauritius had to win. During my training, my shoulder was getting worse and worse. I was getting stronger, but my serve was hurting me badly. I also had to play in tournaments consistently, and that was no fun; to be hurt and beat by 16-year-olds. The weight of all of this started to burn me out. I had surgery to correct my SLAP tear but unfortunately I didn't get any better. My shoulder continued to be painful and my serve was very weak. Not good enough to play at a high level. I didn't make it to the Olympic tryouts, but I cheered my teammates on. In the end, Mauritius didn't make it to the Olympics.

It was a bitter end to a grueling 10-year tennis career, but just beyond the horizon was the start of a new adventure: bouldering. I started traveling with Dave and other friends to new and exotic climbing locations, like Joe's Valley, Utah. Well, maybe not new or exotic, but exciting all the same! As I became immersed in the climbing community, one thing became quickly apparent: I had to either embrace the dirtbag lifestyle or start looking for a career. I was on a student visa that only allowed me to stay in the US one year after I graduated. I knew I didn't want to go back to Australia, and I also knew that I didn't want to be a translator or a language teacher. But I did know that I loved training, moving and climbing. Inspired by what Dave had done for so many climbers, I decided to study exercise science and become a strength coach myself. I didn't know much about training, except that I had trained a lot! Coaching, though, was nothing new, I continued to coach tennis until I left Denver.

Under the guidance of Dave Wahl and my advisor at Metropolitan State University, Dr. Joe Quatrocchi, I learned as much as I could about training, health and fitness. These two guys gave me different perspectives on training; whether teaching folks who have never worked out before or training elite athletes. I loved this so much, that I went on to pursue a Masters degree in Human Movement. I realized that I had so much to learn, and that I would try to get as much experience as I could while I was in school. I worked at a few laboratories at the University of Colorado Boulder. I helped out in the Neuroscience lab, learning about stress and performance. I also did a few semesters in the Motor Control lab, learning about how people learn, what motivates them and how best to deliver information to perform a task. I loved this whole process. When I graduated, I got a job at my Alma Mater. Dr. Quatrocchi saw my passion for learning and knew how much work I had put into getting to that point. I was hired on as Adjunct Faculty and started teaching other students about health and fitness. I was also working at Movement Climbing and Fitness, as well as the Denver Bouldering Club, as a performance coach, teaching climbers how to get stronger, develop skills and take their climbing to the next level. I had the opportunity to train many other types of outdoor athletes, such as mountaineers, triathletes, skydivers and ultra runners. During this time, I learned so much from all of them.

My personal development was also thriving. I continued to train with Dave, bouldered a ton and started climbing higher grades. I thought I would give it a go at competition bouldering. This meant that I had to train a minimum of 15 hours per week, plus work. It was a challenge I was willing to take. I had only been bouldering for about three years before doing my first professional comp and was recovering from a torn ACL the year prior.

I competed in the ABS nationals. At the time, there weren't as many females competing, so I did well. Not well enough to be in top 10, but good enough to get a small sponsorship with Scarpa. Scarpa didn't just sponsor me for climbing, because I honestly wasn't as good as my peers, but they sponsored me because of my love and passion for the sport. I started a blog, GirlBeta.com, that encouraged more females to boulder and train so that we could all crush! I put free training videos up and "beta" videos of climbs. The site was so well known that I got more sponsors for the site. I competed again in the ABS Nationals the year after and did slightly better, but then tore my ACL in the other leg. I focused my training on my upper body and learned more about how to recover from big injuries. It actually served me well when it came to injury prevention training, as well as rehab training for my clients. I bounced back again from this injury and competed in my last big competition; the regional comp in Brisbane, Australia. I decided to compete while I was down there visiting my family. I did really well and was invited to compete in the national competition, however, I was on my way back to the US. Had I participated in this competition, I would have had the opportunity to compete in a World Cup. I still regret not doing it to this day.

All of this personal experience was so fulfilling and amazing. I was amped to continue training, but the opportunities in Denver weren't there. I had done what I could and hit a ceiling. That's when I got an offer from Vertical World Seattle to develop their fitness program. I saw this as an amazing opportunity to create something relatively new in the climbing industry: to create a full strength and conditioning program for outdoor athletes. Seattle wasn't just filled with climbing enthusiasts; it was filled with people who did numerous outdoor activities on a regular basis. For example, a person might have a collective background in skiing, alpine climbing, cycling, ultra running and kayaking. How do I best serve such a diverse athletic population through training? It had to be a program that developed strength, as well as skills, that intersected all sports.

Creating this program was partially experimental and also heavily research based. I took information from many different conventional strength and conditioning protocols and blended it with some old school training I had read about from climbers. I had also adopted many philosophies from my mentor Dave Wahl and continued researching the best way to train, in a short amount of time, that developed skills, strength, fitness, prevented injuries, increased mobility and was fun! My evolution as a coach was definitely from conventional strength and conditioning to more progressive, bodyweight skills training. Based on my experience, I know that some training best serves some athletes better than others. This is where the art of training comes in: being able to give something to someone that completely works for them, and then giving something similar and it absolutely not working for someone else. Working through this and figuring out ways to best train individual people is why I love what I do.

HOW TO USE THIS BOOK

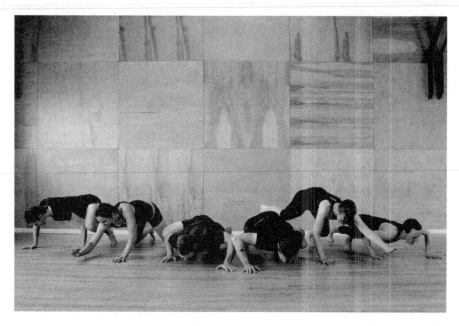

As you peruse this book, you will notice that each exercise has a written description, a photo description, and for some, a video demonstration.

For some of the exercises you will see an icon like this "▇◀" which means that there is an accompanying video on YouTube. Go to SimpleStrengthBook.com to view the Youtube playlist or type this link into your web browser: http://bit.ly/1K2zVIM

The photos are meant to show you a snap shot of each "phase" of the movement. Below is an example of what the photos will show.

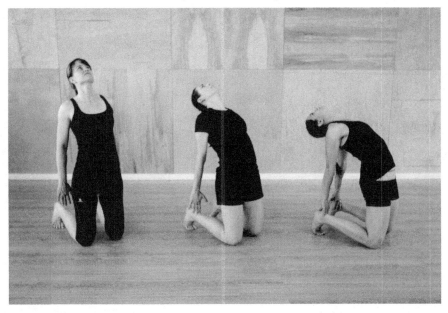

The first model on the left is showing the first position of the movement, the next model shows the intermediate position, and the last model is showing the final position.

Some photos may just show a different perspective of the position described.

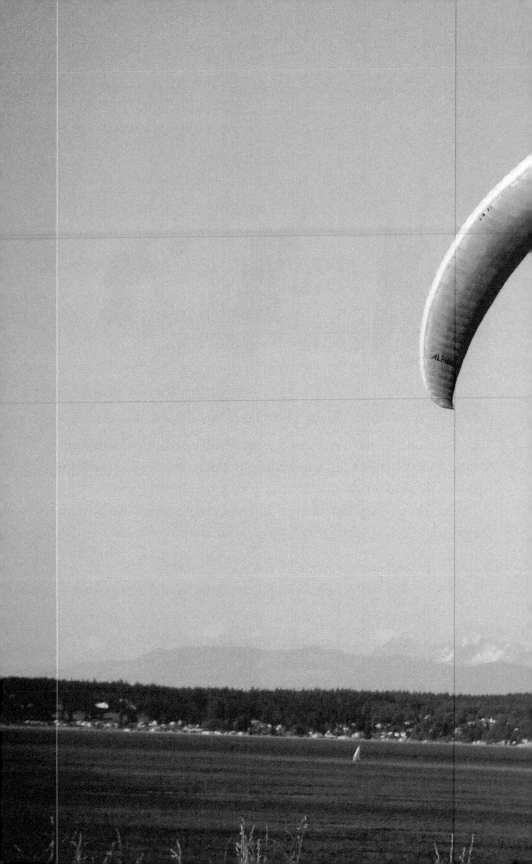

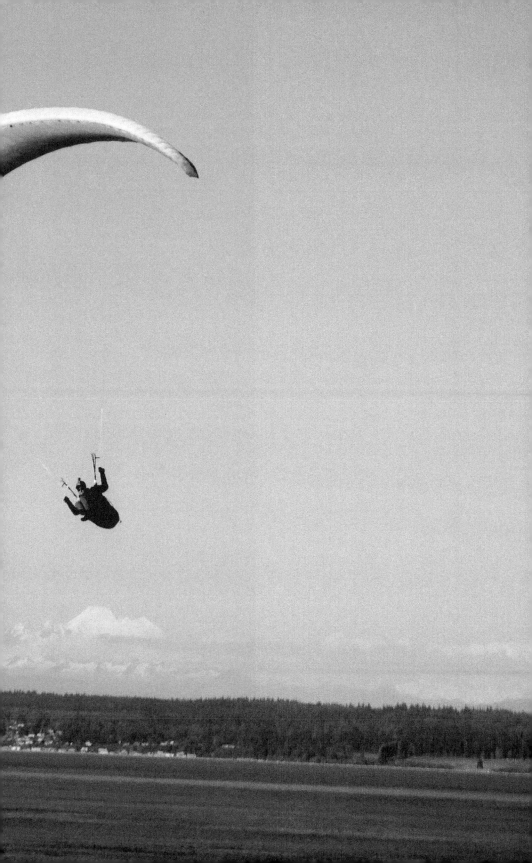

2

SECTION TWO

BASIC PRINCIPLES

What Do Outdoor Athletes Need?

Outdoor athletes spend a ton of time "doing" their activity or sport, and usually on the weekends. And if they do train, they are training the aerobic system, when they have spare time, using protocols that they found on the internet. Self-coaching is a big part of outdoor culture, where coaches aren't often used to make programs more efficient, measure weaknesses and assess strengths. Outdoor athletes should consider hiring coaches to evaluate movement, design individual programs and to make training more efficient and useful. In addition, if an athlete is only focusing on the aerobic side of training, they are missing a huge chunk of the athletic equation. To increase performance and decrease risk of injury, athletes should train all the facets of movement: balance, strength, endurance, power, coordination and mobility. In this book, I will cover mostly strength, balance and mobility. You can also apply these concepts to power and coordination.

Why Do I Emphasize Bodyweight?

Because it is always there. You always have your bodyweight. You don't need fancy equipment, or even need to be dressed, to use your bodyweight. You can wake up, be in your PJs and bust out some back bends. You can also use your bodyweight while you are traveling. Sure, fancy equipment allows you to do exercise while sitting, isolating muscles, without having to control your bodyweight to balance, or even focus on alignment. But this isn't functional, or realistic. Outdoor athletes continually push their bodies to the limits, making awkward moves, hauling more than just their bodyweight and needing a strong instinct to survive. When our brains are activated by these demands, we fall back on our normal movement patterns. And, if your training comes from exercise equipment that doesn't allow full freedom of movement, you will be inefficient; compensating in areas that are already strong, reaffirming your weaknesses, and eventually causing you to break down.

What is Strength?

"Strength is a Skill" - Pavel Tsatsouline

Muscular strength is the ability of a muscle to exert a maximal or near maximal force against an object. It could also be defined as the quantity of muscles being recruited, as well as the ability of the nervous system to appropriately activate the right muscles during exertion. If the nerves aren't doing their job, your muscles won't activate. The brain sends messages down through your nerves to activate the muscles to move.

It's a common misconception that the size of a muscle defines how strong it is. I bet there are some muscle bound people who probably can't touch their toes, or do a simple back bend. What is the use? Our society is so focused on how we look and not how we perform. I'd be more impressed with someone doing a one-arm chin up than a 300-pound bench press (I do believe that bench press is a good test for upper body strength, but not a good way to train). Plus, doing a chin up is way more practical. Unless you are a firefighter, or in the military, you will never find yourself stuck under 300 pounds, with a fixed structure under your back, and needing to lift that object off of yourself. Which brings me to another point about muscle size and function: the more muscular you are, the heavier you will become, which is not what most outdoor athletes need. They need to be fast, light and agile. There is no use for extra muscle mass to haul around. This is where training your nervous system comes into play. Strength training is usually split up into two different areas, hypertrophy and max strength. These are two ways to train the muscle for strength. This book will cover the later, max strength, which is more functional and practical for outdoor athletes.

High Tension to Increase Strength

Since you have your bodyweight to work with, you can manipulate intensity by changing positions and controlling momentum. In every move that is shown in this book, you are required to come in and out of tension. Increasing tension will increase the amount of muscles recruited by the nervous system. The more nerves involved, the stronger you will become. A nice byproduct is that you increase muscle tone, making you look more defined. You also need to be able to come out of tension to relax the body, and then ease back into tension to reactivate those muscles, which grooves the neural patterns from your brain to your muscles.

Perfect Practice

"Perfect practice makes perfect" - Kelley Starrett

One of my favorite quotes about this matter is from Gray Cook, the creator of the Functional Movement Screen. He says,

"If movement is dysfunctional, all things built on that dysfunction might be flawed, compromised or predisposed to risk even if disguised by acceptable levels of skill or performance. Poor movement patterns demonstrate increased injury risk with activity, but good movement patterns don't guarantee reduced injury risk. Once fundamental movement is managed, other factors like strength, endurance, coordination and acquisition of skill also play a role in prevention. Movement comes first."

This means, that when you do move, you need to focus and move with pure intention. Don't rush through the work, and make small adjustments as needed. To know if you are moving well, the best strategy is to video yourself doing each exercise, analyze it and then move again. Be your own critic and judge. With each exercise you do in this book, do it with intention, video yourself, and don't get bogged down with the number of reps and sets. Execute all exercises well and stop before you get to failure. Stop if you feel like your form is being compromised. Setting a time limit is the best approach to staying focused.

Basic Rules

Before starting any program, or learning any new skill it's important to remember my basic rules:

#1 Be Kind to Yourself
#2 No Negative Self-Talk
#3 Leave your Ego at the Door and Try Hard!

Without these rules, you may hold yourself back. You may not reach your goals because you're stuck on "results" rather than the process.

Progression

Progression and patience are additional ingredients you need to master a skill. Slow and steady, maximizing the movement for all it is worth, and analyzing your movement, will all pay big dividends in the long-term process of movement. Making technique and skill a priority will develop your neuromuscular system and result in what most people call "muscle memory." The grooves form from your brain to your muscle, establishing a solid pathway. If for some reason you take a break, and come back to the skill later, you will still have the techniques to pull off the moves, even though you may lack the 'strength' to do it. So take your time, don't rush through the progressions and always come back to the basics.

You Are Your Own Project

You should treat your body like a project. It is your only body, and you only get one. Eating clean, moving right, and thinking clearly will all help you find flow. And having flow is happiness. Being in the zone, doing the things you love and performing how you want to perform is what we all want. Treat yourself right, take your time and build yourself into a machine; a beast that can move fluidly, think clearly and is masterful.

WHY I CHOSE THESE EXERCISES

These exercises can be done anywhere, anytime, with no special environment or clothing needed. The workouts can be quick and concise or as long and complicated as you want them to be. However, the movements themselves are considered complex. They are not so simple to execute and require a lot of attention to detail and discipline. Anyone can 'get through it', but that doesn't make it challenging or meaningful. I want these exercises to be meaningful to you. People want to move and feel free. And if you practice these movements, you will get that feeling.

These exercises are also fun do to. You can get a group of friends and do them together. Having partners critique you, spot you and motivate you is a great way to work out.

These movements are, in my opinion, basic human movements. Our bodies were meant to move. Moving freely in all directions, through all ranges of motion.

The more you practice these exercises, the more functional they will become. In the beginning, the technique should be challenging. The technique requires you to think about each intricate movement and your alignment. But once you've practiced technique, it becomes intuition and you just move. That's when you go on to something more challenging. These movements that you practice create patterns in your nervous system. These patterns will cross over into other more functional movements, such as lifting up grocery bags from the ground, putting big boxes away on the top shelf of your closet, moving furniture and so on. I hear a lot of people saying that they tweaked their back picking up the laundry basket. THIS SHOULDN'T HAPPEN! It's because these simple patterns aren't there. The patterns that *are* embedded are sitting positions and linear movement positions. Twisting, turning and core control aren't all consistent parts of your everyday sitting lives. That's why it is imperative to move in directions and push your body in ways that are hard, so that your life can be easier.

These fundamental movements are also seen in many outdoor sports. Squatting, pushing and bending back are all parts of athleticism. In rock climbing, you have to twist and bend to see handholds, where to place gear, or to move through a roof climb. You also have to get your feet high to move and push up with your legs, and you have to push with your arms to climb dihedrals, or scramble. All of these movements form a foundation of skill, and later in this book, I give numerous variations to these exercises to challenge you.

CKC vs OKC

Before I move on to talking about the crossover of skill that these movements offer, I want to make sure that you understand that there is no such thing as *isolated exercise*. If you voluntarily move one body part, you are affecting another part of your body no matter if it's on an exercise machine or not. This is because the body is connected with a web of fascia. This fascia is what covers all cells, organs, bones, muscles, the brain and the skin. With each movement, you are involuntarily affecting or using another part of your body. But, the degree in which you affect or recruit other parts of the body comes down to the *Chain of Movement*.

Every time you move in every day life, you are likely performing *Closed Kinetic Chain* (CKC) movements. If you go to the gym and use machines, these are considered *Open Kinetic Chain* (OKC) movements. CKC is defined as having the foot or hand in a fixed position as you move, whereas in OKC, the foot and hand move freely. OKC exercises are often what most people think of when we say *isolated* exercise. It usually targets one muscle group or joint. CKC exercises usually require the whole body to execute the movement. *Simple Strength* covers CKC movements because you are aiming for more functionality and maximum recruitment from other parts of the body.

The Crossover of Squats
- Great for hiking, skiing, climbing, cycling.
- Benefits any lower body movement that requires good body position.
- The squat variations primarily work the glutes and quads, but there is so much more going on in this movement. It works on external rotation of the femur, ankle stability and mobility, spinal strength and endurance. If done very well, you can work on your posture and core control too.

The Crossover of Push ups
- Great for scrambling and climbing.
- Also great for opposition training to any pulling that you might do as an ice climber, rock climber and kayaker.
- Primarily works the pectoral and tricep muscles. When done correctly and intently, the core should start to burn. You can also see the transfer of the "plank" position to any strong standing positions.

The Crossover of Back Bends
- Good training for awkward movements in climbing and kayaking.
- Great for oppositional training.
- Improves spinal health and mobility.
- Primarily works the posterior chain of the spinal erectors, glutes and hamstrings. Also works shoulder, thoracic, and neck mobility.
- Back bending also offers good spinal health and the ability to 'open' up after being in a hunched position most of the day.

TECHNIQUE AND MOVEMENT

The more you commit to moving well, the fitter you will become, which means you will be able to do more work.

As you train, it is imperative to focus on good technique and taking your time to feel the movement. Nothing good can come from rushed movement that looks janky, out of control and has no tension. Your intention should be your own movement. Get into the zone, block out distractions and focus. If you do this a few times, you start to appreciate the movement. You learn more about the movement, how certain joints feel, and how much muscle needs to be activated.

Be Disciplined. Master your own movement.

Video Record Your Movement

Being aware of your movement can be tough when you don't know how it is supposed to feel. The best is to watch an example of it, and then video yourself doing the same thing. Be critical, does it look similar? Make sure to look at the position of your back, feet and hands. These can give you clues into what your movement is doing. If your feet are turning out during the movement, it probably means that your knees are buckling in, or if your shoulders are rounding forward, it probably means that your spine isn't straight. Pay close attention. It may take a few times to view the movement first, execute it, then critique it. Once you critique it, try again, but better.

Movement Improvement

How do you know you are getting better at the movement? Firstly, you will feel stronger. Secondly, you will know by testing. You should retest a measurement and retest by video recording. You can do both or either. This will make sure that you aren't just getting strong, but that you are getting strong in the correct way.

Flow

Look at an exercise you want to do. Watch the video a few times. You can stand in front of a mirror. Take a few deep breaths and imagine yourself completely alone, working on your craft. Increase your tension, and start to move. Take note of small adjustments. Take your time. Make corrections. Repeat as necessary. Remember, there is no negative self-talk and no ego here. Only movement.

Cascade Effect of Good movement

Good intention of movement = increased awareness of movement = learning = better alignment = better movement = movement efficiency = skill development = increased capacity to do more work = FIT.

Cascade Effect of Poor Movement

Minimal intention = poor awareness = poor posture = poor movement and movement control = poor efficiency = limited mobility = GETTING OLDER BEFORE YOUR TIME.

PAIN

You know the saying, "no pain, no gain?" Well, I say that's a load of doodoo. But I guess it's also how you interpret the saying. For too long, it's been meant to encourage athletes to push through injuries and pain, and if you stop because of pain that you would be thought of as a wuss.

Pain Present? Address it!

The kind of pain that you want to push towards or push through is the muscle burn. Even here, you have to be careful. If your muscles are burning, they are saying that you are getting fatigued. What happens when you get fatigued? You lose form. And then what happens when you lose form? You increase your risk of injury through bad movement patterns.

When to Push Through the Burn

Whenever you want. It's up to you. Each of us has a different tolerance for pain, that's why it's important to assess it as it's happening. If you are to the point of burning, you know the risks. Are you in a controlled position? Is there risk of dropping weights? Is there risk of moving poorly? It's really up to you.

But What About Real Pain?

Oh, you are talking about pain pain. The pain that makes you want to run away. Like I said before, if there is pain present, address it. The only pain that should be pushed through is the burning feeling. Otherwise, all other pain needs to be addressed. Stop, analyze the pain: is it going to be worse if you keep working through it? Is it getting worse?

Current Injuries

If you are about to start this program or try any of the exercises for the first time and you have a current injury, I would highly recommend going to see a rehab specialist if you haven't already done so. Take these exercises to them and ask if you can perform any of them without making your injury worse. If you don't know, ask! It's not worth hurting yourself more, and then taking a whole bunch of time off because you just wanted to push through it.

List of Possible Pains

- Muscle burning: Good
- Any other type of burning: Bad
- Cracking with no pain: Fine
- Popping with no pain: Fine
- Cracking and popping with pain: Bad
- Tweakiness: Fair - Assess where needed
- Aches: Bad
- Shooting: Bad
- Pinching: Bad

- Stabbing: Hmmm...this could be a muscle cramp. Assess where needed.

Address the Pain During Your Workout. Don't Push Through It.

If you keep feeling pain after you stop, and it's persistent, consider seeing a professional rehab specialist. And see a specialist that works with athletes.

Ice

I have been going back and forth about ice therapy. I still don't know what the right answer is. Here are the theories out there right now:

1. Use ice immediately to bring down inflammation after an acute injury.
2. Don't use ice after an acute injury. Rather, wait a few days. Initially, use electrodes and heat to draw out inflammation and circulate blood into the injured area.
3. Use ice for pain management.
4. Use heat to circulate blood a few days after injury.
5. Use ice on chronic injuries to control inflammation.
6. Use heat on chronic injuries to circulate blood.
7. Use both ice and heat on chronic injuries.

Ice and Heat for Recovery

I use different methods depending on where the pain is. I only ice for about a minute, or as long as I can stand it. For me, I only use ice on my finger joints if they are inflamed after a long climbing session. I mostly use movement and massage for inflamed joints, and for my fingers I use a rice bucket. Heat is amazing for blood circulation and works great for nighttime therapy while you sleep. There is research on ice and heat therapy for recovery, and I know many endurance athletes who use an ice bath, or water that is around 55 degrees, to recover. There is some evidence that this helps to recover muscles and joints before the next training session.

A rice bucket is a regular bucket filled with uncooked rice. Then you place your hands in the rice and move in specific directions such are side to side, forward and back, full rotations, squeezing the rice, and extending the fingers. The rice provides appropriate resistance for rehab. The rice can also be replaced with dried beans, or other types of rice or lentils to change the resistance on the hands and fingers.

Movement as Medicine

Movement is the best medicine. That's what this whole book is about. If you are hurting, explore ranges of motion that don't hurt, and keep the joints and tissues moving. This will help speed recovery and ensure that your joints don't get stuck.

Taking Time Off

If it hurts to do the things you want to do, then you have to stop doing those things. Maybe choose something that doesn't hurt, but can keep you active. I train a ton of climbers, and many get finger injuries because of strange handholds. This is a horrible thing when it does happen, and none of them know what to do. While I don't think taking time off is the best answer, I also don't think pushing through the pain will help either. Find positions or movements that don't hurt. I like the help of tape to increase my awareness of the area, as well as to protect it from any further damage. Using rice bucket therapy and hand putty works well too. Either way, just keep moving!

BENEFITS FOR OUTDOOR ATHLETES

Outdoor athletes are multifaceted, usually doing several spokes in the wheel of activities. Each spoke represents an activity that will eventually help them reach their goal. For example, alpinists must learn the skills to hike, rock climb, ice climb, manage rope and make fast decisions, as well as condition for several aspects of their ascent such as altitude, weather, carrying heavy loads, and the list goes on. The point is, they don't just do *one* thing, they do many things. And training usually is *doing* the things. The only time training might become a part of the regime is during the off season of your sport or when the terrain isn't available. But, to stay in shape, to progress and continually reach goals, it's imperative to train, and training should develop a base of strength and conditioning.

In the words of Steve House and Scott Johnston, from their book "Training for the New Alpinism," "*Structured coaching in competitive sports, and recently in sport climbing and bouldering, helps athletes learn how to train.*" Structured coaching is not seen in many outdoor sports. You should be spending a majority of your time *doing* the sports, and structuring how much and when to do these makes a very big difference in performance. It can be the make it or break it of reaching a goal.

Strength training, as seen in this book, is just one small part of the overall training program. This was designed so that you can do these exercises quickly, with minimal equipment and perform each well. These are considered 'strength' exercises, but could also be done in conjunction with conditioning. (Note, these exercises are not a replacement for more sport-specific training. In order to excel at your sport, you need to put the time in to develop the specific skills of your sport. These exercises are intended to help guide your overall movement)

These exercises will help the outdoor athlete build a base of strength and incorporate movements that are seen in all sports. The outcome from doing these exercises will be to become a well-rounded athlete. Doing these moves correctly will help you become more fluid in other movements.

Injury prevention is another benefit of strength training. As your movement awareness improves, you increase your control in possibly dangerous situations. However, I will say, that if you train more and are very physically active, you walk the fine line of staying healthy and being injured. The more you do, the more likely you are to get injured. However, doing these exercises can bounce you back quickly from injury.

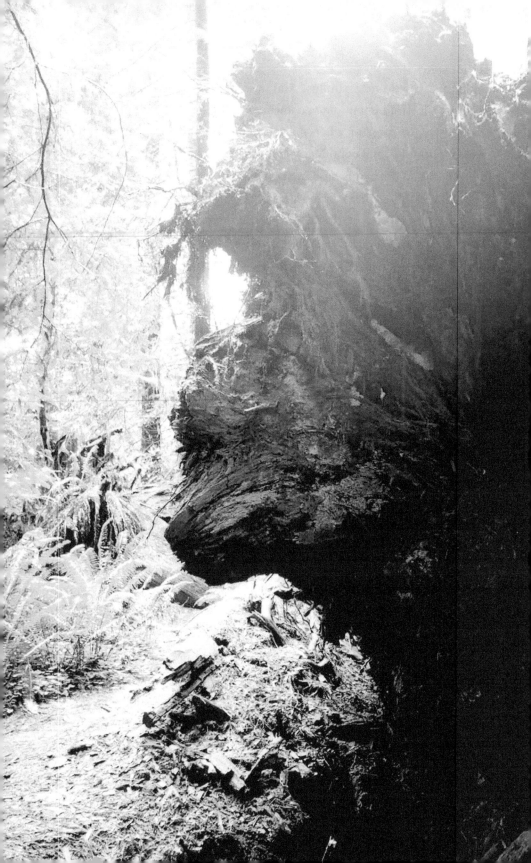

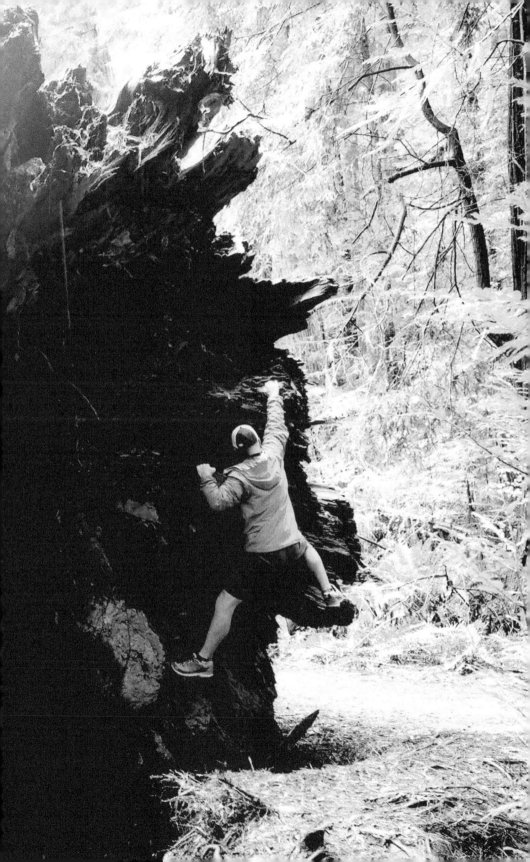

3

SECTION THREE

SETTING GOALS

Before I go on to explaining what goals are and how to set them, I want you to answer the first two questions below. This will help you determine your goals.

#1. Why Are YOU Training?

Before you start training, you need to figure out what you are training for. I think more often than not, you start a program and don't think about why or how you are going to go about it. I train because I want to continue moving and learning new ways to move.

#2. How Will You Fit Training into Your Schedule?

This is also important to think about when starting any training program. I hope that I will help you figure out how these exercises will apply to your sport, but you have to be willing to take action and make a plan to stay committed.

How to Set a Goal

What are goals good for? Goals are good for keeping us consistent, motivated and being accountable to ourselves. The types of goals you set will help you become successful. Here are some great tips I got from the

TED article "The Science of Setting Goals" written by Kelly McGonigal. She shares four tips to help us be successful.

1. "Choose a goal that matters, not just an easy win."

There are easy, manageable goals that can be obtained everyday, and I'll talk about these later in the Creating Habits section. But the overall goal, as McGonigal explains, should be meaningful, something that will inspire you each day. Here are a few goals from my clients: Ascend and ski down Mt. Rainier in under 10hrs, eat healthy and become fit so that cancer won't come back.

2. "Focus on the process, not the outcome."

This is where the cliché, "*it's the journey, not the destination*" can be used. And this couldn't be more pertinent for outdoor athletes. It's the nature of outdoor sports to rely or work around weather and environmental conditions. Or whether you are healthy enough or have trained enough to complete an activity. In reality, you can't control the end result. you can continue to push forward, to take risks and keep the end goal in your sights —that's what you have control over.

3. "Frame your goals positively."

Instead of making negatively worded goals, such as, "I don't want to be lazy anymore," you should spin it into something positive so that your brain will naturally want to pursue it. Rather, say, "I want to workout 10 minutes a day to become stronger."

4. "Prepare for failure (in a good way)."

It is inevitable that you will run into roadblocks. The most important thing is to not punish yourself for it. Remember my 'rules' at the beginning of this book? "Be Kind to yourself and no negative self-talk!" Failures will happen, and each failure is just a step closer to success. But this will only happen if you plan for failures and acknowledge them and move on.

Motivation

Goals can be a great help for getting you motivated. Motivation is what keeps you going on the bad days. It's what drives you. That's why it is so important to figure out why you are training and to set meaningful goals. For most outdoor athletes, you have time sensitive goals, usually an ascent of a mountain, or doing a race. They can also be considered more grandiose, "dreaming big." These kinds of motivations are called external or extrinsic motivations because they are derived from outside of us. And usually, when we are done with one goal, we move onto the next, or, never actually accomplish the goal. Big goals are really great for powering through seasons, and I'm sure, as an outdoor athlete, you have a ton of energy and motivation to accomplish them. But there is a negative to this; it's not sustainable and could eventually lead to burn out.

There is another more sustainable way of approaching and creating goals, and that's with internal motivation. Also known as intrinsic motivation, it is what comes from inside of us. We don't need punishment or reward to reach a goal. It is usually the process of achieving the goal that makes us feel a certain way and makes us who we are. I think this is why we love being outside, doing incredible things in nature. We want to feel the chill on our skin and feel empowered by what we are accomplishing. These types of feelings remind us each day why we do what we do.

We need both types of motivation to reach a goal. And to reach a goal, you need to create a habit around it. That is what I will talk about in the next section.

HABIT BUILDING

Creating Habits

After you set your goals, you have to find time to fit these exercises into your busy schedule. I know that it is difficult for outdoor athletes to find the time outside of their longer workouts to do more strength-based work and cross training, but with these simple habit strategies, you can quickly add these exercises into your daily life.

> *"We are what we repeatedly do. Excellence then, is not an act, but a habit" - Aristotle*

One of my favorite bloggers of 'Habit' is James Clear. I have used some of his ideas and implemented them into my own life the last few years. Here are some strategies that you can use to start integrating these simple exercises into each day, so that you can stay strong, develop good movement and crush your goals!

1. *"Develop a ritual to make starting easier."*
Habits are done day in and day out. They are also 'started' day in and day out. You don't have to think about starting to brush your teeth, or starting the coffee, you just do it. But for a new habit, it's the starting that makes it challenging. There are two ways to start a ritual: "stack" your exercise habit on top of a current habit, or set a schedule for yourself.

Stacking the exercise habit on top of a current habit:

After/Before [CURRENT HABIT], I will [NEW HABIT].

- After I brew my morning coffee, I will do four Shrimp Squats
- Before checking my email, I will do five A-Frame Push Ups

It's a great hack to do if you want to fit these exercises into the day and don't have time to do a full workout. This method is effective because you already have one habit dialed in, and you are just linking your new habit it.

Scheduling the exercise habit:

During the next week, I will exercise on [DAY] at [TIME OF DAY] at/in [PLACE]

In order to write this book, I had to schedule out specific times in the week to sit down and write, because I wasn't able to fit writing in at the same time each day. I don't have a consistent work schedule; I work evenings some days and mornings the other days. So for me, this was a winning method.

2. *"Start with an exercise that is ridiculously easy to accomplish."*

> *"Start with something that is so easy you can't say no."* - Leo Babauta

I love this hack. I tell all my clients this because it has been so successful in developing new habits. For me, running seems to be a habit I can't stick to. So I say, "I'm just going to run for 5 minutes." Sometimes it really is 5 minutes, but more often than not, I run for more time.

For these exercises in the book, I suggest starting with 1-2 minutes for one exercise. That's it.

3. *"Focus on the habit first and the results later."*

This goes back to making grandiose goals and process goals. If you focus too much on the results that you will get from the goal, you probably won't stick to the habit. Usually, this is because the, "ah screw it" language comes in. In general, it is more important to not miss workouts in the first few months than it is to see progress. Consistency will eventually lead to improvement and success.

> *"Objects in motion tend to stay in motion"* - Newton's First Law of Motion

Now that you have come up with some goals, know why you train and how you will fit these exercises into your schedule so that it becomes a habit, you are ready to start thinking about the training plan and how exercises will progress. I will talk about how the conventional training plan is set up and then later talk about how you can use practice rather than a strict plan to get stronger.

HOW CONVENTIONAL TRAINING IS DIVIDED

Setting up a training plan can be a complicated and detail-oriented task, especially for strength and conditioning coaches, who design plans for individuals and teams. It's important that strength coaches follow protocols, to make sure that all elements of training are covered in a timely manner and to gain the maximum results for their athletes.

To give you a better idea of how training is broken down, I will explain to you what periodization is, and explain what each element is.

What is Periodization

It is a training cycle or series of cycles. One cycle consists of a set of phases to develop an athlete without burning out while maximizing the athlete's performance potential. There are many forms of periodization, but in this book I give an example of the basic periodization model (Matveyev's Basic Model). This model has four phases. It starts with a *basic preparatory* phase, then goes on to a *stabilization and strength* phase, then an *event* phase and then ending in a *recovery* phase. This is one cycle. You repeat this cycle over and over. Sometimes the cycle will change depending on whether you need more advanced protocols or not. Each phase lasts around 4-8 weeks. Some might be longer or shorter, depending on the athlete's training experience. You can apply this model to any type of training you want to do. In the Programs chapter, I give you an example of how to apply this plan to the bodyweight exercises described in this book.

Periodization and Why Coaches Do It

Because coaches don't want their athletes to get overuse injuries, and to avoid plateaus and burn out. The system is setup so that an athlete can go through peaks and valleys, days of higher intensity and lower intensity training sessions. This is usually spread out over months of training. Coaches also don't prescribe the same exercise over an extended period of time. They usually change the exercise type, intensity, and volume over time. Also, in general, an athlete's career looks something like peaks and valleys, where performance is what undulates up and down. Athletes don't always have good days. In fact, athletes mostly have okay days and bad days. You train for the good days. Because your performance undulates like this, your program must also be designed this way.

The First Phase: Basic Preparation

In my opinion, this phase is considered the learning phase. This is where you might introduce new exercises and learn how to do each one properly. The second part of the prep phase is building a base of fitness, getting used to exercise volume and getting into good habits. If you can get through this phase, you are setting yourself up for success to finish the program.

The Second Phase: Strength and Stabilization

This is where you make the movements harder. You progress from simpler movements to more complex ones. The reps and sets also vary. In the strength phase, we bring down the repetition and focus more on the difficulty of the task, making it as difficult as possible.

There are two ways to develop strength: one is called *hypertrophy*, the second is *neuromuscular* development. Hypertrophy is seen as increasing muscle size to increase strength, whereas in neuromuscular development, you are increasing the amount of motor neurons, the arrangement of motor neurons, and the pattern of how the nerve impulse is coming to the muscle. The more motor neurons attached to the muscle, the more muscle is recruited when you perform an exercise. The technique in which you perform the exercise is very important because it dictates the pattern of how the muscle is recruited, known as *motor control*. In this book I am primarily interested in neuromuscular development, and to show you how to do this. For outdoor athletes, it is imperative to focus on this because hypertrophy training just adds weight to the body. In general, the lighter you are, the easier it will be to carry yourself up the mountain, or the rock. For mountaineers, alpinists, or backcountry skiers, when you are ascending, you have to carry your own weight. If you can increase strength without gaining muscle mass, you will have an advantage over those who train for hypertrophy.

Nerve Signaling

The *motor unit* consists of the motor neuron and all of the muscle cells it innervates. When a nerve signal is sent down from the brain, all of the muscle's fibers/cells connected to the motor neuron are asked to contract. This pathway is called the *motor pattern*. The number of motor units per muscle can vary depending on what function the muscle is involved in. For example, fine motor control of the eye has been observed as having one motor neuron per 100 muscles fibers. Whereas in the thigh, where a large amount of force is produced, and where fine motor movements are not necessary, there could be one neuron per 2,000 muscle fibers. Motor units are not considered static structures. Motor units adapt to a variety of neural, hormonal and metabolic stimuli resulting from functional demands and neuromuscular activity patterns. Which means, the more stimuli, the more motor units.

Motor Unit Recruitment

The neuromuscular system can increase the contraction force of a muscle through two basic mechanisms; recruitment and rate coding. More motor units will be recruited as the force or intensity of the muscle contraction increases. Rate coding is the frequency of the motor units being recruited. The more a muscle is being asked to contract, the more force is increased.

The Third Phase: Event

When I develop programs for outdoor athletes, usually it's more pertinent to enter into what is known as a "power endurance" phase. To lead up to an event, other athletes usually go through a power development phase, which is designed to mimic the event that you will be participating in as closely as possible. It's the phase where exercises become more sport specific. When you look at soccer, basketball and tennis, this is where you see force development needed for skills such as sprinting across the field, hitting a forehand and quickly changing directions. But for the outdoor athlete, in most cases, you are concerned with doing forceful movements over and over and over again, for a very long period of time. This is why it is called power endurance.

These first three phases form the classic pyramid illustration. The bottom of the pyramid is the preparation phase, the middle is the strength and stabilization phase, and the top is the event phase. When you reach the top, you are ready to do your event, or for the date of event that you have been training for. You are able to execute your event. You are forming this base so that you can build on top of it; the longer and wider you can build this base, the taller you can make the pyramid.

The Fourth Phase: Rest and Recovery

This is the last phase of the periodization model: the recovery phase. This is possibly the most important phase for professional athletes.

Recovery

Recovery is quite different from rest days. Recovery can be changing up your activity after several months. For example, most professional athletes take three months off from their sport to recover. They aren't being lazy during this time, though. They are still moving, doing other things. But, for the mind and body to take a break from the sport is a great idea, something we should all employ.

Usually, after the recovery phase, the cycle starts again. Most elite athletes go through two major training cycles a year. For most outdoor athletes, you have several seasons that you are training for. And it might not be just two seasons. It is beyond the scope of this book to talk more about how training cycles can be manipulated to keep an athlete at their peak for longer, but it is something to consider when designing a program, or when you are thinking of hiring a coach. But also consider taking time off and doing something that is different than your usual activities.

Rest Days

I'm not a proponent of taking rest days. You can continue to move every day, doing different things each day. But, it is very individual. If you have a problem with overtraining, you should rest every other day. If you are new to working out or training, you should take a few days off each week, and limit your training days to no more than three days in a row. But, if you are used to heavier workloads, you are going to be okay with taking one rest day, if that, each week.

Varying the Intensity within Your Program

It's important to workout at different intensities each day. If you do high intensity every day, it will lead to fatigue that you can't recover from. Doing high intensity work, a few times a week, in addition to whatever your sport is good enough, unless you are getting paid to be an athlete, then you might need to dedicate most of your life to training. See the Programs section to see how I recommend splitting up intensity days.

You have just learned about the four phases of conventional training. Next I will talk about how progression will help you build a foundation of strength, when you should progress and how you know you are progressing.

PROGRESSION

Learning is a process; it takes time and patience. That's why it's so important to use progression when starting anything new or revisiting something familiar. Progression also ensures that you don't get injured, that you aren't skipping over technique basics, and allows for more refined motor control.

When you start something new you have to work your way up. If you can't perform these exercises yet, it just means you haven't developed the appropriate foundation of strength and coordination.

Building a Strong Foundation

You have to focus on building your foundation of strength, mobility and coordination. Creating this strong foundation will help you easily build more complexities onto your basic skills. This is key for maintaining skills and developing future skills.

Going Back to the Basics

This was something I learned from playing competitive tennis. Going back to the basics helps to re-focus, remember what's important and develop basic patterns if you feel like you've lost them somewhere along the way. It's fun to come back to the basic stuff and realize how much you really have progressed.

Don't Skip Ahead

Try not to skip ahead to more complex exercises. Go through the sequences of exercises, test yourself, ask, are you ready to move on? Be truthful about where you currently are. Attempting to make shortcuts usually ends up in setbacks.

Not skipping over levels and focusing on quality is essential for outdoor sports. This applies to learning how to rock climb, using correct systems for alpine climbing, or implementing the correct exiting strategies for kayaking. But often, if you skip over levels for any of these, the results are fatal. TAKE YOUR TIME!

Quality vs. Quantity

> *"Quality practice of fundamental skills over time leads to higher level performance"* - Ryan Hurst, Gold Medal Bodies

Every time you practice a skill, you need to focus your full attention on it because you need to apply quality to the practice. You can't expect to become a master of movement just by watching a few videos. Practice Practice Practice! And in the words of Kelley Starrett, *"Practice makes Permanent."*

Accountability

Surround yourself by those who have been in the same position, who encourage you or inspire you, or who have the same goals as you. This will help you stay on track, stay accountable and be truthful. If you would like further help on your journey, you can always sign up for my *Modus Athletica Online Training*.

Test Retest

Always check in with your own technique. The best way is to video yourself. I'd say retest every two weeks, especially if you decide to go down the 'practice ' route instead of programming. If you feel that your technique looks good, and you've earned the gold to move onto the next progression, do it.

Be Your Own Judge

Take progress notes, save the videos each week and look back at them. See how far you have come. Often, you fail to remember where you started, and don't recognize how far you really have come.

Progression to Ensure Lasting Enjoyment
Enjoy the process, take your time and focus. This will set you up to continue to enjoy the exercises, and keep you going on this movement journey.

Progression, Practice and Training go hand-in-hand when developing skills. The next section will help you understand the difference between training and practice, and help you decide which route to take to develop your skills.

PRACTICE

Practice so that you can move better.

What Makes Practice Different From Training?
Both will help you increase your strength. And strength building should be the ultimate goal for training or practice, because that's what is going to give you your biggest bang for your buck when improving your outdoor skills though cross training.

So how is it different? Practice is more mindful; it's more focused. Essentially, you are slowing your movement down to feel how your body moves, and you assess how good your own movement is. The end result of practice is building skill.

What are skills?
A skill is like riding a bike. You will always remember how to ride a bike once you have learned how to do it. You are developing the motor patterns that tell you how to move appropriately and efficiently. That's what practice is meant for, to build these motor patterns, so that you can remember how to do them, even after you have taken some time off. You can be sure that once you come back from time off, that you will be able to do it well.

Practicing movement also helps you use your current strength more appropriately. Maybe you are super strong but don't have great coordination, and that's okay! Hopefully at the end of this book, when you implement these exercises, you will learn how important coordination, strength, mobility and flexibility are when bringing these all together to master your skills.

Movement in humans and other animals is made up of many different factors: the slow and the fast, the conscious and the non-conscious, the neuronal and the muscular. Some of these factors, like reflexes, are heavily genetically determined and show little, if any, adaptability. On the other hand, many of our movements change over time as a result of practice and learning. These movements tend to differ from purely reflexive movements in both their complexity (e.g., there are many more moving parts) and their adaptability (e.g., the details of the movement can be adjusted to fit a specific context). Often, we refer to these learned movements as "skills" and in a general sense, we may think of skill, "as the ability to do something well." More academically, we can define a skill as the ability to produce an outcome with the highest degree of certainty and lowest amount of time and/or energy.

This definition of a skill is quite useful and forces us to consider skills, and especially motor skills in a different way. We might normally think about skill purely as the neural-side of the equation: controlling the body in a skillful way. That line of thinking, however, quickly gets us into trouble, because it is no good having a nervous system that "knows" how to perform a movement if the movement requires a certain minimum amount of strength or power. Thus, a skill can be the combination of both our brain (the controller) and the body (effector) and we need both in almost all skillful behaviors. Certainly, the skill of chess has less of a musculoskeletal component than the skill of shot-put, but in both cases, the more skillful person is the one who can reliability produce a given outcome with less time and/or energy. In a research lab, we might be interested in adapting the brain or the body to better understand how these complementary parts work in isolation, but in almost all natural activities the brain and the body will be adapting together to produced skilled behaviors. - Keith Lohse, PhD

When you practice, technique should be your number one priority. When you go through all the exercises, focus on technique. In the *Naked Warrior*, Pavel Tsatsouline talks about some basic practice principles to get stronger through bodyweight exercises. I have included some of his ideas with some of mine to come up with a solid recipe for practice.

1. **Focus**. Block everything else out.
2. **Low Reps**. Keep the sets and reps low. This equates to increasing max strength. But of course, each rep needs to be challenging enough to build strength.
3. **Staying Fresh**. At the end of your sessions, you should always feel like you could do more. If you go to failure, you are teaching yourself to fail and how to be tired, not how to be strong and move well.
4. **Practice Daily**. In order to get better, you need to do these exercises every day. Doing it once or twice a week will only slightly increase your strength, but by doing these daily, you will see larger gains in strength. If you do practice daily, try to focus on two exercises that are opposing, like one upper body and one lower body exercise. Doing too many exercises in one day will overcrowd your nervous system and you may end up not learning the movement at all. If you do want to do other exercises, keep the volume and complexity down. The two exercises that you chose should be the main focus.
5. **Vary the Exercises**. When you do this, vary the exercises over time, not on the same day. And don't do the same exercise every time you practice. Try different types of movement over weeks and months.
6. **Build Slowly**. Progress and test.

How Do You Know When to Move on to a More Difficult or Complex Exercise?

This is where testing is really important. You must take video and be critical of your own movement. Maybe you have been working on something for a few weeks and still haven't mastered it: keep pursuing the same difficulty of exercises. Don't push ahead. Be patient, stick with it.

Once you feel like you have made progress and you are moving well, you can move on. For some of the exercises I have listed, I have placed targets to aim for before moving on to the next progression. Once you do move on, and you have done a lot of different exercises and you are doing it really well, you can always come back to some that you really enjoy. This is what helps you continue your practice, and stay on your path.

Training vs. Practice

In training you usually use reps and sets to determine how much you are doing and it determines your progression. But in practice you use feeling of the movement and execution. To stay focused in practice, you can set time limits to practice a move. Remember, you don't want to go to failure. And you want to stay fresh at the end of the practice. There is no set program, just doing what you enjoy doing right now. And do this every day.

Now that you understand the theory of training and practice, it's time to turn your strength into a skill. In the next chapter, I will show you how to execute all the moves properly, so that you will have the tools to move correctly.

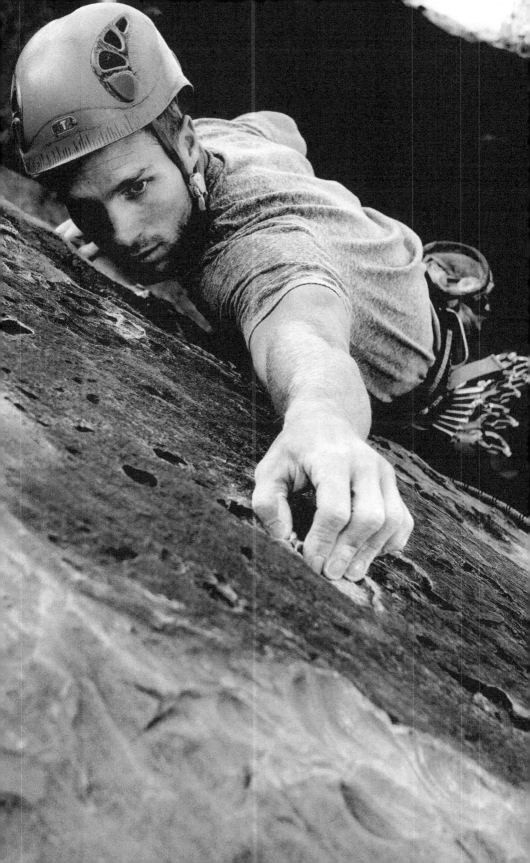

4

SECTION FOUR

TENSION AND TECHNIQUE

READ THIS FIRST before moving on to the exercises. In order to bring forth your best technique, I have given you some really great cues to keep in mind when executing the exercises.

#1 Create Tension

In Pavel Tsatsouline's *Naked Warrior* he stresses the importance of tension. This is an amazing cue to have because it doesn't just help you during these exercises; it helps during more difficult moves in your sport. The more tension you create, the more strength you will have to execute the move. So as you go through each of these exercises, create tension throughout your whole body and see the difference it makes.

> *"Tension = force"* - Pavel Tsatsouline

Tensing the Abs

As you are about to set up for each exercise, see if you can tense up your abs. Doing this will increase the intensity of the muscle contraction you will focus on. By contracting your abs, it creates a corset, a rigid cylinder to support your spine that is very, very important in moving well and creating stability. *No Floppy Fish!*

HOW TO: Your abs should draw your sternum and pubic bone toward each other in a straight line. Keep the abs flat. Brace your abs as if you are expecting a punch in the stomach. Another way to feel this tension is to lay on your back with the legs at 90 degrees. Press your lower back into the floor. Notice the pressure in your abs when you do this. This should be the tension you create when you brace.

Tensing the Glutes
This is setting up your largest engine in your body to ignite and propel the movement.

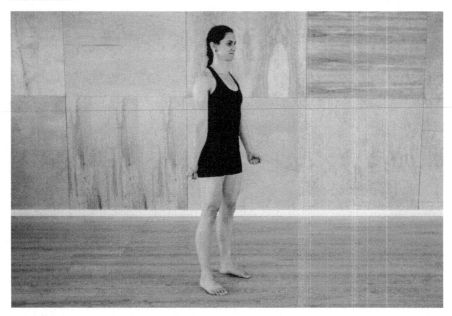

HOW TO: Pinch a quarter between your butt cheeks. Your pelvis should tilt slightly up (Posterior Tilt), and this will happen when you tense your abs up too. You want to tense both abs and glutes at the same time.

How Much Tension is Enough?
It depends on how difficult the move is. If you find it challenging, you need to increase your tension as much as you can, so that your strength will increase in these movements. If you are breezing through an exercise

with good form, you can choose to do it with less tension, requiring less energy to execute the move.

#2 Static Stomp

This is a great technique to create power from tough positions. The stomping feeling can be used through the heels of your foot in the squat and through the heels of your palms in the push up. Stomping creates a reactive force between the body part and the ground. The greater the reaction force, the greater the power you have to move the body.

HOW TO: At the beginning of the movement, you want to start with this feeling of stomping through the ground. Many yogis use this in mountain pose to help them feel more grounded. You are going to use this to generate more power. Before you move, stomp through your heels. As you move down into the squat or pistol, feel yourself "pulling" toward the ground. Before you ascend back to standing, "push" through the ground, and then stand. Feel the tension that is created when doing this. Think about pushing the ground away from you as you do a squat or a push-up. In a squat and back bend, this actually increases glute activation. In the push-up, it increases lat activation.

#3 The Corkscrew

This is a critical technique cue to get the shoulder and hip joints into a powerful position for movement. You may have seen this technique in action in the "Perfect Push-up" handles. They are tapping into a shoulder position that will recruit the lats while you push, as well as increase the reactive force during the movement. I will show you how to do this without the handles.

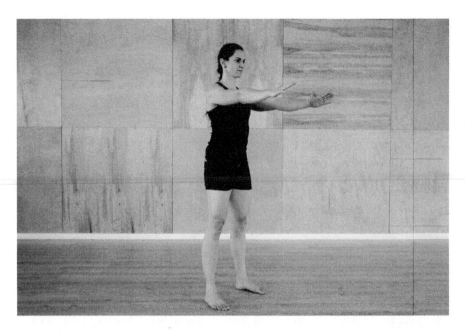

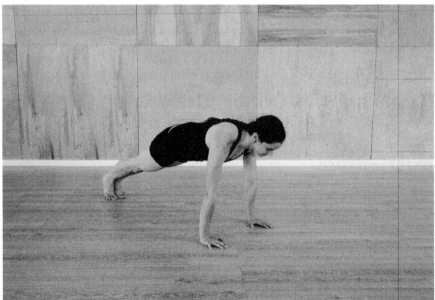

HOW TO: Think about spiral tension in the arms and legs. For the push-up, to get into the right position by standing up straight, then grab a bar with your hands and try to snap the bar in half. This is spiral tension. When you are executing the push-up, without moving your hands, try to rotate your arms out. The elbow pits should rotate out. As you move through this motion, especially in the bottom position, really exaggerate this cue. This goes for the squat and back bend position as well. Spiral tension should be created up from the feet through to the thighs.

Things to Avoid

No bouncing! Never ever. Try to never do this, you are just robbing yourself of strength and possibly hurting yourself.

Neck Flexion. Try to keep your neck neutral during all movement. If the spine is staying straight, then keep the neck straight with it, if the spine is bending, then your neck can bend with it.

ADVANCED TECHNIQUES

Isometrics

Stopping at certain angles in the squat and push-up will increase your strength quickly, but it is much more difficult to execute. You can try isometrics in the squat or pistol by moving down to 90 degrees in the knee, hold for a few seconds, come back up. You can also execute this in the push-up, by going down to 90 degrees in the elbows, and holding here. You can try going down to 90 degrees and holding, go all the way down and holding with tension, and back up to 90 degrees and holding, then all the way back up.

Isometrics to Strengthen Weak Spots

Pick a variation that you are comfortable with, use assistance if you need to, and try the isometric technique. Stop where you feel weak, and increase your tension. Pay attention to your body, what do you have to do to increase tension?

Quick strength

For all the moves, including the back bend, you can gain quick strength by holding the bottom position of each for a few seconds when you execute.

It is similar to isometrics, but rather you are focusing on the end position rather than the 90-degree position. Hold the bottom position for a few seconds, under tension, and then come back out.

Dead Starts

At the bottom position of the push-up, the pistol or squat, you start in a relaxed position and then add tension before ascending. This is great for training the weak links in your movement.

TECHNIQUES FOR THE PUSH-UP, SQUAT AND BACK BEND

PUSH-UP

1. Toes together.
2. Hands shoulder width apart, index and middle finger pointing forward.
3. Form a solid plank position. Increase tension here. You should feel a ton of power in your body.
4. Focus your attention on the armpit, increase tension here. Think of the Corkscrew.
5. Shoulders must stay low. Otherwise you disconnect the armpit from the torso.
6. "Pull" yourself down to the ground, keeping elbows tight to your sides and head in front of fingers.
7. Before you ascend, feel yourself push the ground away.
8. Push from the armpit rather than from the shoulder.

Breathe: Inhale on the way down, hold, and then exhale as you push up.

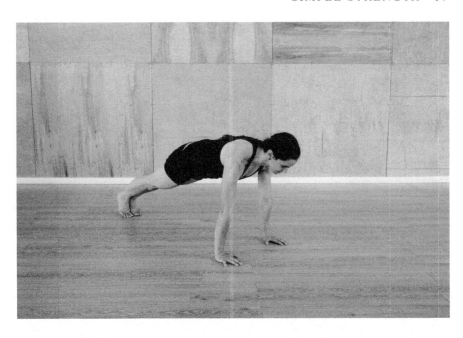

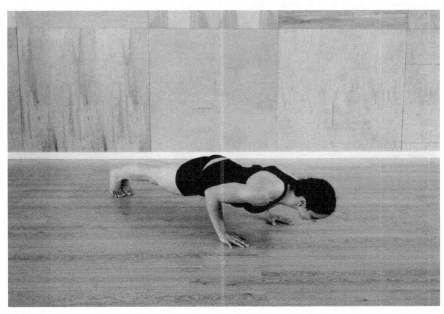

SQUAT

1. Find a good stance with your feet. I usually like just wider than my shoulders.
2. Keep toes pointing straight forward.
3. Stand with tension; abs and glutes tight.
4. Head of the arm rotated back into its socket. Corkscrew.
5. "Pull" yourself down, keeping your chest up and neck neutral with the spine.
6. Knees should push out to the side. Don't let the knees fall in!
7. Go down as far as you can, keeping heels pushing through the ground, and spine straight.
8. Before ascending, stomp the heels and squeeze the glutes to push you up to the start position.

Breathe: Inhale on the way down, hold, and then exhale as you push up.

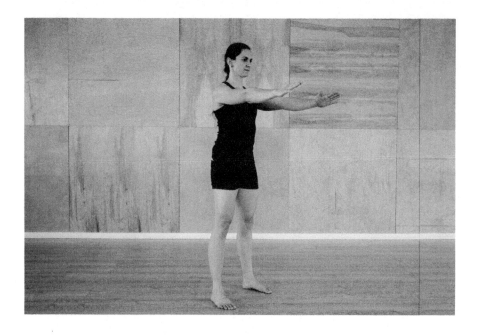

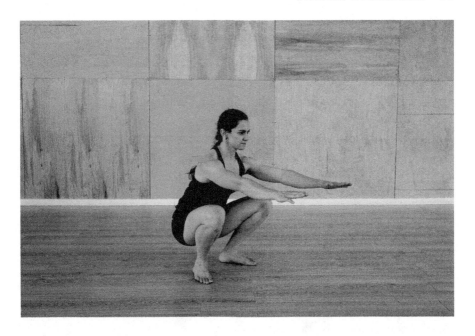

BACK BEND

In the back bend, you want the spine to be mobile, so the sequence of tension will be slightly different compared to what you read above. Don't try this without doing the preparation bends first. The back bend is an amazing spinal strength exercise and hip opener, but it is quite challenging and should be approached with caution.

1. Tense up from the ground, pressing your heels into the ground, and follow tension up through your body.
2. Your thighs should be engaged, "zipping up" your kneecaps (Kneecaps draw upward).
3. Try to force some separation between your thighs without moving the feet.
4. Lead with the arms going back, fingers pointing back. Keep abs slightly tense.
5. Look back at your hands, and try to find the ground.
6. Keep leading with your eyes to the ground.
7. Don't let your glutes squeeze too much, instead try to tilt the pubic bone upward.

8. Reach back slowly until your hands make contact with the ground.
9. Press your heels into the ground.

Breathe. Try to relax your breath. Constant breathing.

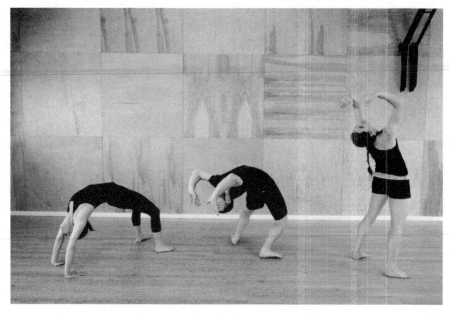

POSTURE AND ALIGNMENT

Body awareness is an important part of improving one's movement. And it all starts with posture and alignment. Once you feel how your body should align, you're more likely to get into this position without having to think about it. Proper alignment should start from the ground up.

Feet are hip width apart, in neutral position, toes facing forward. Knees should align with toes. If you were looking sideways at your position, your hip sockets should line up with the ankles. The "sit bones" (ishial tuberosities), should be pointing straight down, creating a posterior pelvic tilt (pubic bone rotates up toward your sternum). The rib cage should float onto of the pelvis, with the sternum positioned just in front of the pubic bone. The shoulder sockets should line up with the hip sockets, which line up with the ankles. And lastly, the head should float on top of the shoulders. Ears would line up with the shoulder sockets.

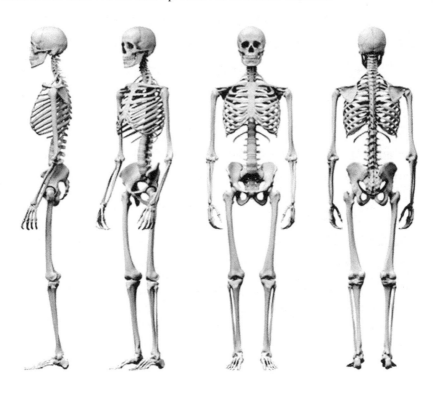

I would consider this a very basic way of describing body alignment; there is so much more to this on an anatomical level.

"Zipping up" for Better Posture

This is an advanced technique used to gain more tension and increasing force during movement. This technique is taught both by Tsatsouline and Starrett. It is also used in many martial arts, to create more body tension, awareness and strength. I would recommend practicing this to improve your standing posture as well as your strength. It will ultimately help you feel how the body should align.

This technique is done in the top positions of the squat, pistol and push-up. Start by tensing the quads and "pulling up" your kneecaps. Now pull the quads up into the groin. Do this to the rest of the thigh muscles, contracting them and pulling them up. Flex your glutes. Everything should be tight and muscles short. You just zipped your lower body up to the hips. Now for the upper body. Continue on to the waist. Create a "rigid cylinder" by tensing your obliques, abs and lats. Keep the cylinder and make sure your abs are flat. Zip all of this down toward your pelvis. Keep your breathing constant and shallow. Breathe from the diaphragm, not the chest. Screw your shoulders into the sockets and really engage the lats. Zip your shoulder blades down towards your pelvis. Tense up the muscles in the upper arms and pull them up into the deltoid. Lastly, gather up your forearm muscles and pull them up to the elbow joint. Once you have this mastered in the start positions, you can try it in the end positions of the push-up, squat and pistol.

Notice how after you are zipped up, everything was pulling you to your core, your center? If the core is strong and stable, it will allow your limbs to move freely. Instead, humans often try to stay strong and stable in the shoulder and hip joints, resulting in "tight" shoulders and hips.

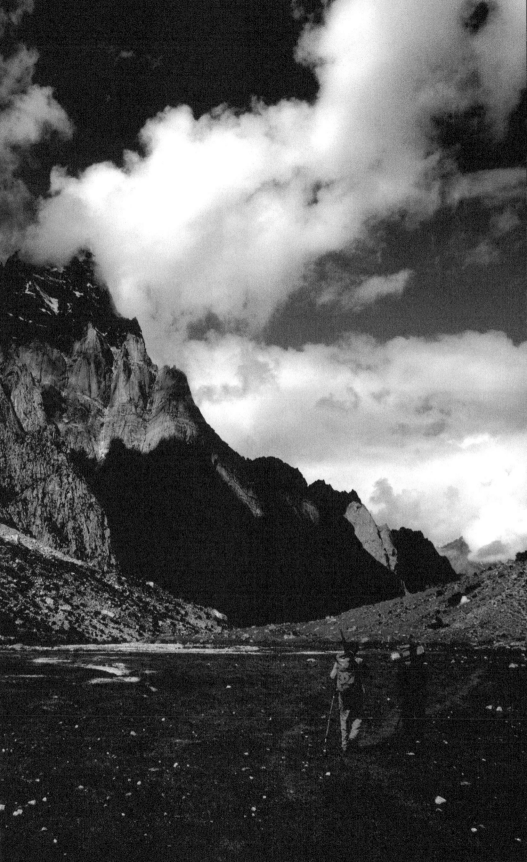

5

SECTION FIVE

TESTING

In order to know where you currently are strength-wise, you can try some of the tests listed below. Each one is meant to precede the next test. Try not to skip progressions, but of course, if your target is to do a pistol, and you have good mobility for the full squat, then start practicing your pistol, even if you haven't passed the tests. BUT, a word of caution, it is better to build up the strength to perform these exercises in conjunction with learning the skill.

PROGRESSION TESTS

BASIC PUSH UP PROGRESSION	#REPS OR TIME
Plank	60s
Wall Push Up	40
Bench Push Up	30
Lower Down to Knee Push Up	25
Push Up	20
Narrow Push Up	10
One Arm Push Up	5-10

BASIC HANDSTAND PROGRESSION	#REPS OR TIME
A-Frame Hold	60s
A-Frame Push Up	5-10
Face the Wall Hold	60s
Handstand	10s

BASIC PISTOL PROGRESSION	#REPS OR TIME
Wall Squat	60s
Assisted 90 Degree Squat	40
Squat to Box	30
Assisted Full Squat	20
Full Squat	30
Feet Together Squat	20
Single Leg Squat from Bench	10
Pistol	5-10

BASIC BACK BEND PROGRESSION	#REPS OR TIME
Superman	30s
Bridge	60s
From the Ground Back Bend	30-60s
Camel	30-60s
Walk Hands Down the Wall	30-60s
Back Bend	30-60s

TEST - RETEST

First, decide which moves and *targets* you want to work on. Now go ahead and video yourself on these moves and targets. Once you have videoed yourself, play it back in slow motion if possible. Play it three times and with each one keep this in mind:

- The first play of the video, look at your lower body. It is doing what it is meant to be doing?

- The second run-through, look at your upper body. How is your spine positioned? And are your shoulders down?
- The third run-through, look at your torso, this will help you see the whole movement. If you don't have this kind of patience, you can look at it once and focus on your torso only. The motion of the torso can tell you a lot about the movement. Now compare your video to either the pictures or video provided in this book. Does it look the same?

Make sure to save all of the videos, put the date on them and share with your friends. I recommend retesting every two weeks.

Getting an Eye for Movement
Here are some tips to help you figure out if your body is moving well.

#1 Look for Alignment. From the ground up, look for lines of movement. Most of the time, the toes and ankles should line up with the hips. The kneecap should be inline with the 3rd toe. In the push-up and squatting movements, the spine should stay neutral without exaggerated curves. Following the line up your body, your shoulders should line up with the hips. Both the hips and shoulders should make horizontal lines, no dipping should occur. Your arms should stay in line with the shoulders. And lastly your neck and head should stay neutral. Don't let your chin jut forward and up, ever.

#2 Look at your Spine. The spine will show immediately if you are leaking power from your movement. Any over curving, flexing and extending, is a sure sign that you are overcompensating somewhere else in the body, or that maybe you lack strength and stability somewhere. The whole back should be relatively flat; this includes the scapulae and the top of the hips. In the squat position, it is imperative to keep the shoulders above the hips, instead of letting your chest fall downward as you squat. You can get a good sense of what this should feel like in the Face the Wall Squat found in the squat exercise section.

Now that you know what to look for in the videos, and you have your target movements chosen, it is time to start moving! In the next section, I will show you how to properly warm up so that your body is ready to move and primes your body to execute the moves properly

.

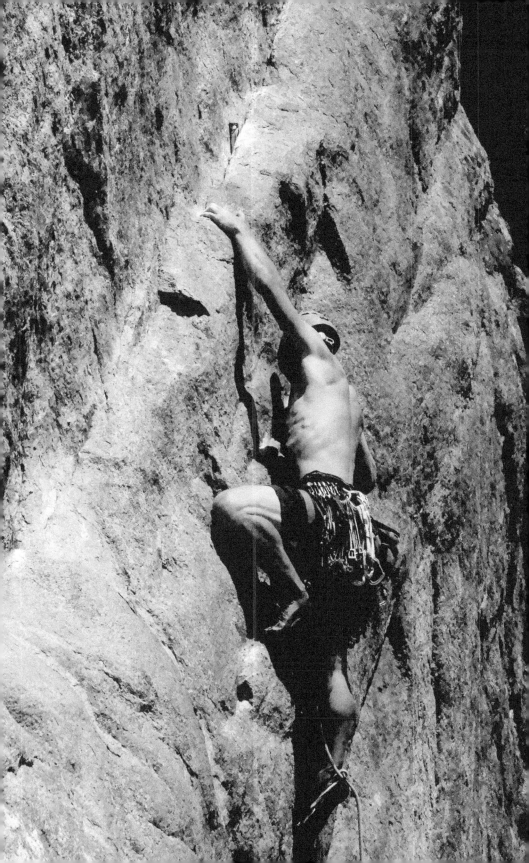

6

SECTION SIX

THE EXERCISES

This next section of the book you will see all of the photos, descriptions and some video demonstrations for the exercises. First you will go through the warm up, then onto the variations. Try each exercise if you like as you read through these sections.

WARM UP

◾️ In this warm up, the primary goal is to prepare the joints for movement. You aren't stretching. You are increasing the range of motion. For each one of the exercises, do 5-10 reps of each or until you start to feel loose. These are just a few exercises I have chosen that will increase the quality of your movement. Feel free to add to this with your own warm-up exercises.

Flip through the next few pages to see the exercises. Don't rush through these movements. They are meant to prime your body for intentional, fluid movement.

ARM ROTATIONS

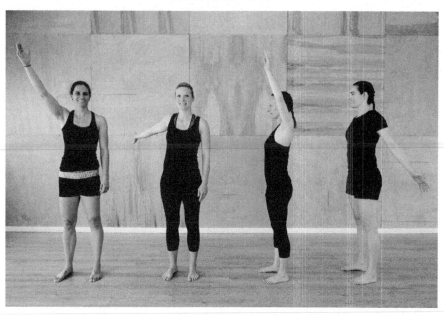

Start standing, rotate one arm in a big circle, with the arm straight. The arm should brush your ear as you circle up. Do both directions of circles with both arms.

SPINE - FORWARD BENDS

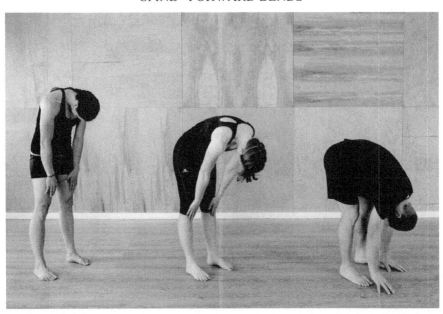

For all of the spinal bends, let your head lead the way, acting as a weight that pulls your body down. Start standing straight with feet shoulder-width apart. Tuck your chin and start pushing each vertebra up to the ceiling as you start to roll your spine forward. Go SLOWLY. Bend your knees as you start to feel your hamstrings stretch. This isn't a hamstring stretch, rather this is to increase articulation of each vertebrae. Come back up slowly, letting your head be the last part to come up.

SPINE - BACKWARD BEND

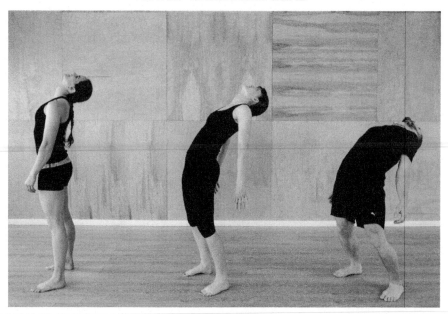

Start standing straight with your feet wider than your hips. Tilt your head back, and SLOWLY bend back. Push each segment of your sternum up to the ceiling. You can bend your knees to increase the bend. Keep your arms relaxed back. Come back up slowly, letting your head be the last part to come up.

SPINE - SIDE BEND

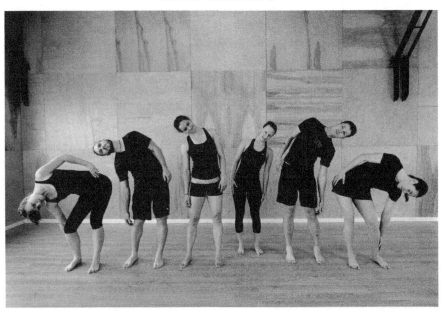

Start standing straight, with your feet as wide as your hips. Bring your ear to your shoulder and start to fall to the side. Keep your arms relaxed. Each vertebra should articulate with the next vertebra. Keep your hips facing forward as you bend. You should feel a deep stretch on the outside of your ribcage. Try to increase this stretch as much as you can. Go down as far as you can, then start to bend your knees to go a bit farther. Go SLOWLY. Come back up slowly, letting your head be the last part to come up. Switch sides.

SPINAL ROTATION

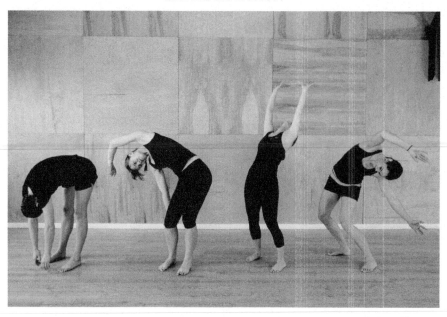

This is a combination of all the spinal bends. Start with the forward bend, this time with feet wider than hips. Go SLOWLY. Now, pretend that there is a stick a few feet above you. Rotate your body to the side into a side bend, then keep rotating until you are in a back bend, trying to keep yourself under this imaginary stick. Keep rotating to the other side and return to the start. Change direction.

PUSH UP PUMP

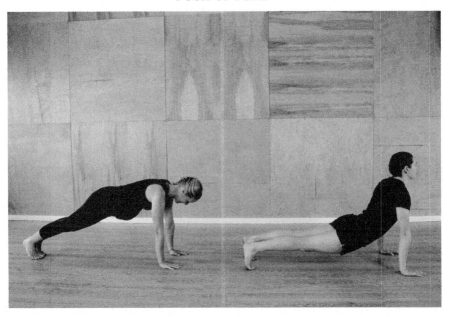

Start in a plank position on your hands. Keep tension. You can either go into a push-up, or skip this. Next go to Up Dog, driving your chest up toward the ceiling and pressing your shoulder blades down. Keep the glutes tight. Push back to A-Frame, pushing your hips up to the ceiling, arms and legs as straight as possible. Return to Plank.

BENT KNEE PLANK

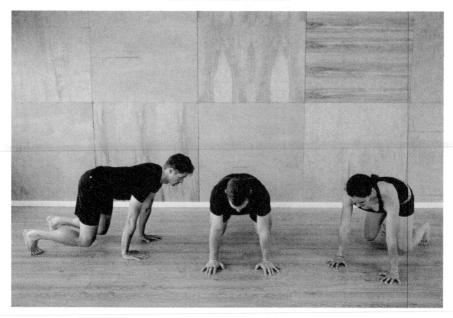

Start with all fours on the ground. Knees under hips and hands under shoulders. Keeping tension, lift your knees a few inches from the ground. Hold this for 10 seconds, then return to the ground.

BEAST CRAWL

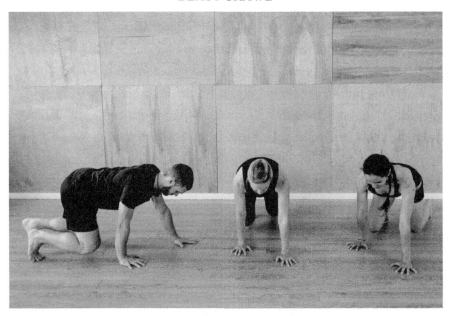

Start the same as for Bent Knee Plank. In the up position, take the opposite hand and opposite foot and move forward only an inch or two. This is a short, slow crawl, not a dynamic big crawl. Take a few steps forward and then try the crawl backward. Keep your knees close to the ground, collarbones lifted, and tension in the torso.

WARM UP WRAP UP

This warm up should take about four minutes. It can be longer if you prefer, working on ranges of motion that you feel stuck in. I love working on the spinal bends. I feel that years of being a competitive tennis player, and only moving in certain directions for hours on end, glued my spine. I have difficulty moving in the grey areas of the spinal bends, transitioning from the side bend to the back bend. It feels quite liberating when I spend some time working on the spine before going onto bigger or more challenging movements.

Next I will show you some of the best variations of the three basic human movements, starting first with the Push Up.

7

SECTION SEVEN

PUSH-UP VARIATIONS AND PROGRESSIONS

Basic Push-Up Progression from the Testing Section

- Plank
- Wall push-up
- Bench push-up
- Not the knee push-up
- Push-up
- Narrow push-up
- One arm push-up

Basic Handstand Progression

- A-Frame Hold
- A-Frame Push-Up
- Face the Wall Hold
- Handstand

Flip through the next few pages to see the variations of the Push Up.

PLANK

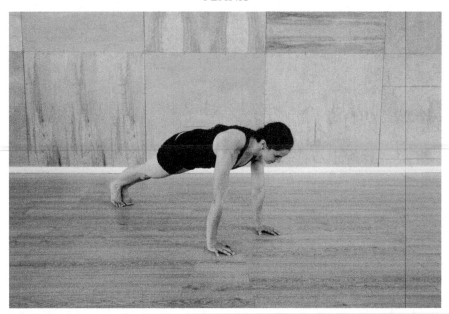

This can be done on the hands or the elbows. For the necessity of working on skills progression, you should do this on your hands. Place hands under shoulders, fingers pointing forward, and big toes touching. Push hard into the ground with the hands, fingers and toes. Increase your tension, everywhere. Think about tension in your armpits, thighs and shins. You should begin to shake if you are doing this correctly. Remember to stop before you start to fail or if your form starts to break down.

WALL PUSH-UP

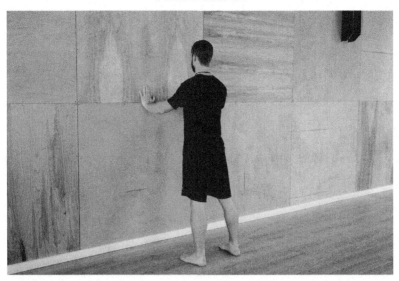

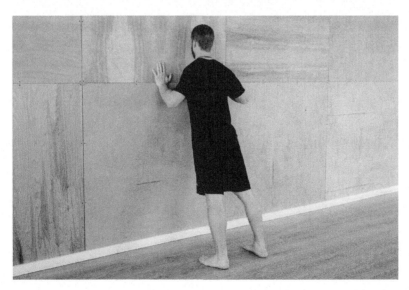

This can be done with hands wider than shoulders or hands shoulder-width apart. This will feel a bit awkward, but do your best. Start in Plank position. Increase tension! Bring yourself to the wall by bending at the elbows, keeping tension in the armpits, not letting your elbows flare out. Go as close to the wall as possible, and push the wall away from you to return to the start. Your heels will come off the ground as your toes act as the fulcrum point.

BENCH PUSH-UP

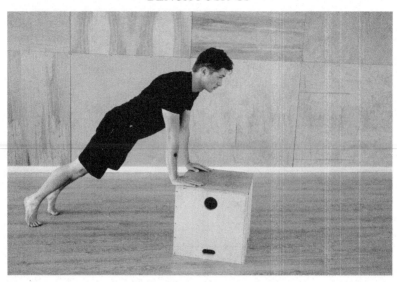

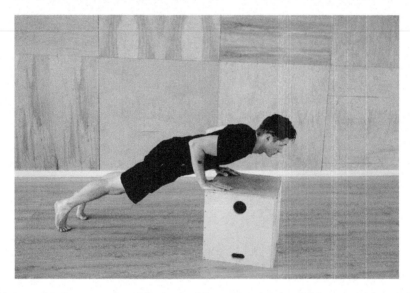

■◀ Start in the amazing Plank position. Hands should be as wide as the shoulders. Pull yourself down toward the bench. Remember tension and armpit pressure. Press the bench away from you. Keep elbows close to your sides and bring your chest as close to the bench as possible without losing form.

NOT THE KNEE PUSH-UP

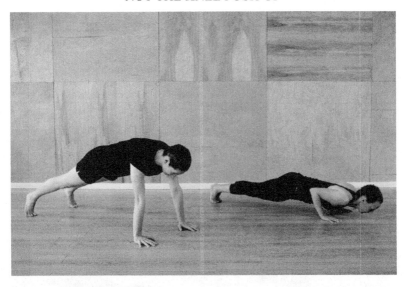

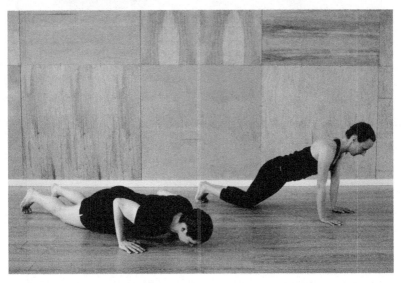

■◀ This is the best variation to work up to a true push-up movement. Start in Plank position. Hands as wide as your shoulders. Tension, tension, tension! As you pull yourself down, keep your head forward of the fingertips. Once you have reached as far as you can go, bring your knees gently to the ground, don't change position of your torso! Then press the ground away from you. At the top, bring the knees back up to start in Plank position. I prefer to do this variation because it mimics the true push up. If you practice the knee push up, it may take much longer to develop the strength to complete the true push up.

PUSH-UP

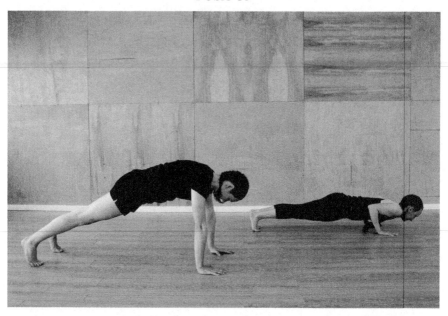

◼◀ Start in Plank position. Increase tension here. Shoulders must stay low, otherwise you disconnect the armpit from the torso. "Pull" yourself down to the ground, keeping elbows tight to your sides, and head in front of fingers. As you ascend, feel yourself push the ground away. Push from the armpit rather than from the shoulder.

DIAMOND PUSH-UP

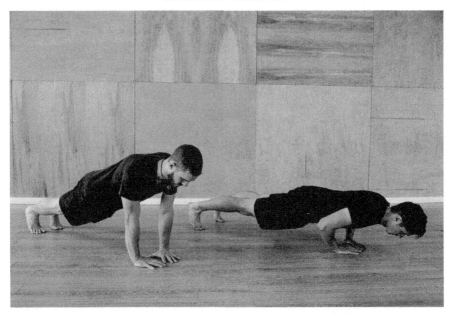

Start as for Push-Up, but with hands close together, making a diamond shape with your index fingers and thumbs of both hands. Keep elbows out to the side. Chest should come down to the hands.

WIDE PUSH-UP

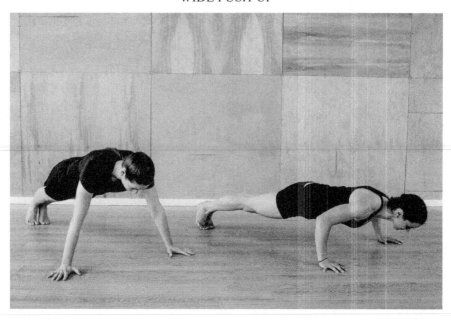

Start as for Push-Up, but hands are much wider than the shoulders so that at the bottom position, your elbows will make a 90-degree angle. Keep head in front of the fingers. Of course, you can work on going even wider with your hands; just make sure your shoulders stay down.

STAGGERED HAND PUSH-UP

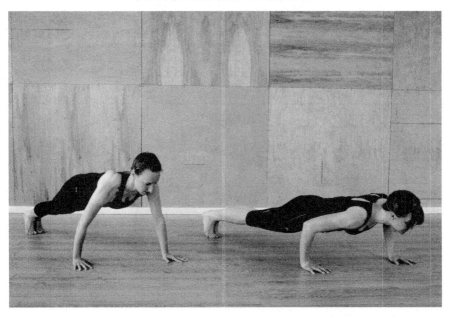

■◀ Start as for Push-Up, but hands are staggered one in front of the shoulder and the other hand behind the shoulder. As you go down, you will notice your top hand's elbow coming out to the side. Don't let it flare out too much.

REVERSE HAND PUSH-UP

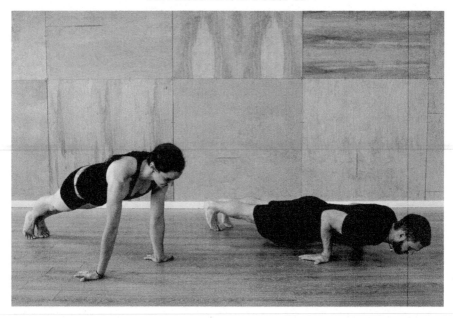

■◀ This is one of my favorite exercises to demonstrate proper push-up technique. Start as for Push-Up, but turn the fingers so that they point back. Elbows stay tight to your sides. This is a great variation if you are working on *planche*. This movement also reinforces good push-up technique.

FIN PUSH-UP

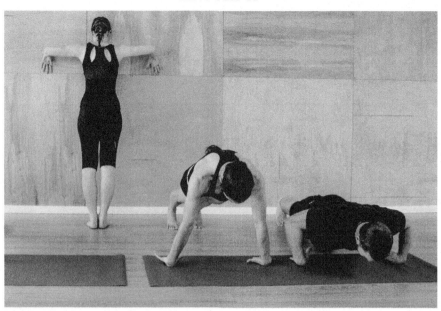

Do this one on a mat to provide cushioning for the wrists. Start as for Push-Up, but flip your hands so that the backs of the hands are on the ground. The pressure should be placed at the top of the wrist. This is a great variation to build up wrist strength. You can also do this on the knees or against the wall to take weight off of the movement.

ONE LEG UP/ONE ARM-UP

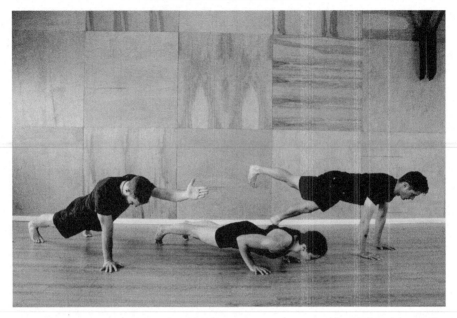

Start as for Push-Up, but at the top, bring one leg up, or one arm up, or both! Keep limbs straight when you bring them up. Don't let your body shift. This is a great conditioning and core exercise.

SPIDER CRAWL

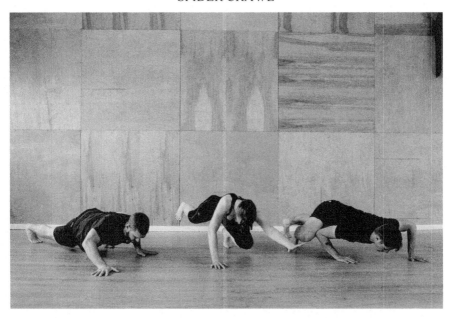

■ This is an amazing movement and so much fun! Start as for Push-Up. One leg and the opposite arm move as far forward as you can. The knee of the leg moving forward should end up touching the elbow. Lower down to the ground. Stay low, and move the opposite side. The goal is to stay as low as you can the whole time.

BEAST CRAWL

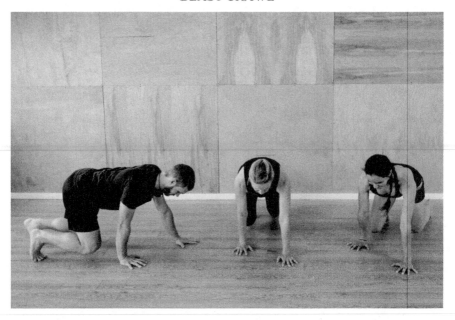

■❮ Start as for Bent Knee Plank in the warm up. In the up position, pick up the opposite hand and foot and crawl forwards only an inch or two. This is a short, slow crawl, not a dynamic big crawl. Take a few steps forwards and then try the crawl backwards. Try to keep your knees close to the ground, collarbones lifted, and tension in the torso. You want to move as if you have a cup of coffee balancing on your lower back.

HINGE PUSH-UP

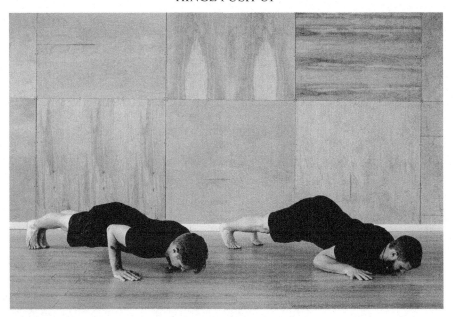

Start as for Push-Up. Lower down into push-up, at the 90-degree mark at your elbow, hinge the elbows down towards the ground and then bring them back up. Return to start position. Keep elbows tight to your sides.

FINGER TIP PUSH-UP

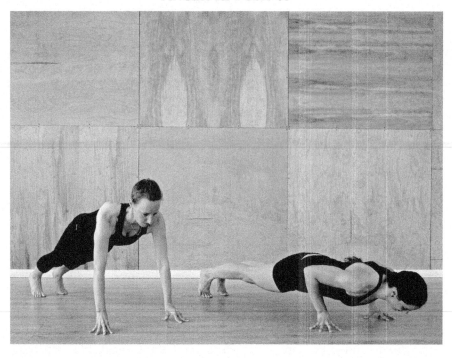

Start as for Push-Up, but the base of each finger will hold up your weight. Great exercise to develop balanced finger strength for climbers.

HANDSTAND PROGRESSIONS

A-FRAME HOLD

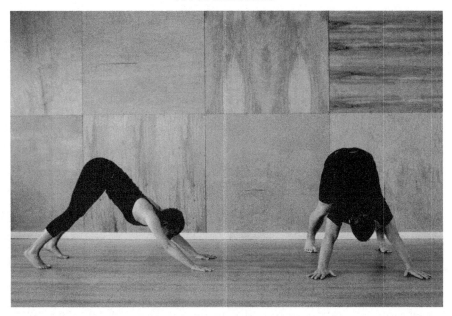

◼ Start as for Plank, but with feet as wide as the hips. Push hips up to the ceiling, making an A shape or pike. Keeps arms and legs as straight as possible. If your hamstrings are over-stretching you can bend your knees. Keeping this position, push away from the ground, engaging the armpit area. Hold this and breathe.

A-FRAME PUSH-UP

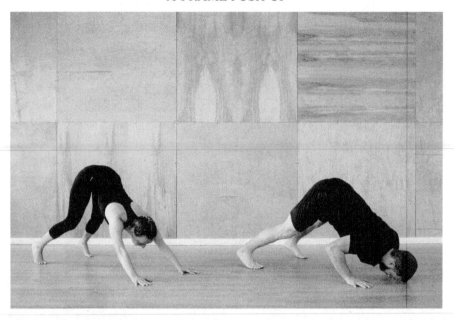

■◖ Start as for A-Frame Hold. With hips up, begin to bend elbows and lower your head down in front of your fingers. Don't let your head touch the ground. Go slowly, otherwise your head may come crashing down. Keep elbows back. Press the ground away as you push back up.

HINDU PUSH-UP

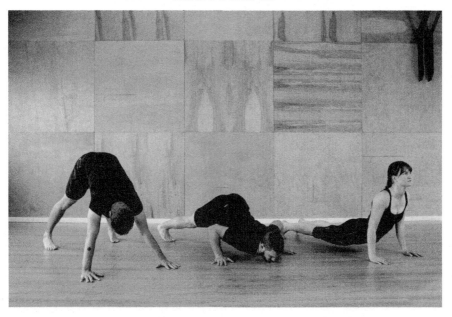

◼◀ Start as for A-Frame Hold. Pretend that there is a stick in front of your shoulders that you need to dive under. Lower your head down toward your hands, trying to slightly brush the ground with your nose. Continue the movement by driving your nose forward and start looking up toward the ceiling. Go up to Up Dog position. From here you can either go to back to A-Frame, or for more of a challenge, reverse the movement.

FACE THE WALL HANDSTAND HOLDS

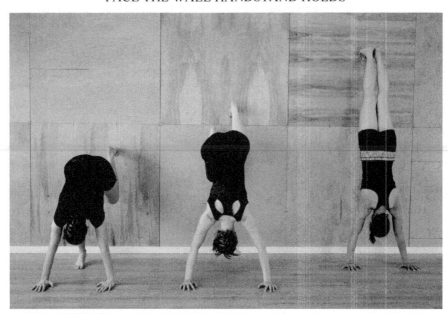

■◀ This is a great progression to work on to get to the true handstand once you have the strength to hold up your bodyweight. Walk your feet up against a wall, and walk your hands in as much as you can. You can start with your legs bent, but try to progress to straight legs and getting as close to the wall as possible. "Press away" from the ground. Keep your body long and tight. Point your toes. For the more break dance style handstand, look down between your hands. Hold this position as long as you can. Breathe.

BUNNY HOPS

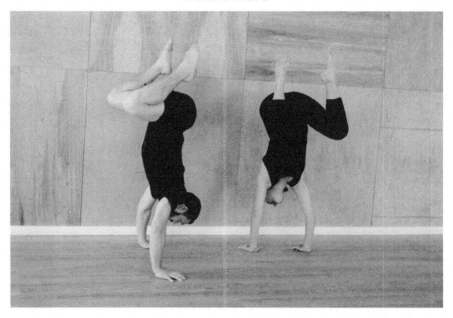

■◀ Do this in front of a wall. Start facing the wall. Place your hands a few inches from the wall. Stay looking at the ground between your hands. Kick up with both feet, tucking the knees to the chest and bringing the heels up to your butt. Try to hold for a second and come back down. This is done for reps or can be done for holds. Great exercise to develop control in the inverted position.

CROW

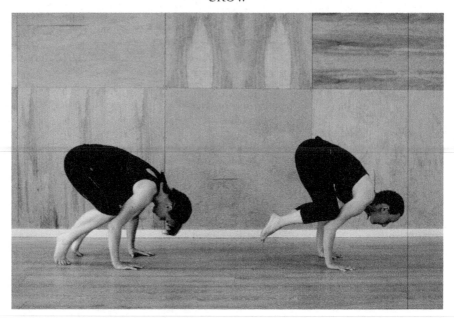

◀ Start on the ground with your hands in a diamond position. Then separate your hands as wide as your shoulders. Bend your elbows. Place your kneecaps on the pits of your triceps. Your feet should still be on the ground. Start shifting your body forward onto your hands. Let your fingers help with stability. There should be a lot of pressure in the fingertips. Drive your body forward slowly, bring one foot off the ground, then, you can try to bring up the other. Hold and breathe.

HANDSTAND

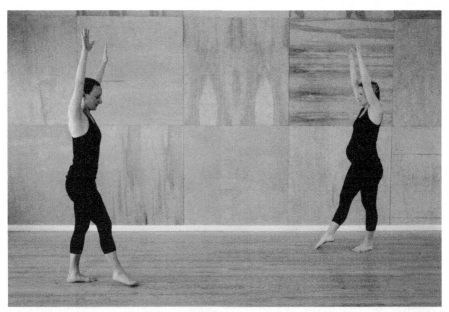

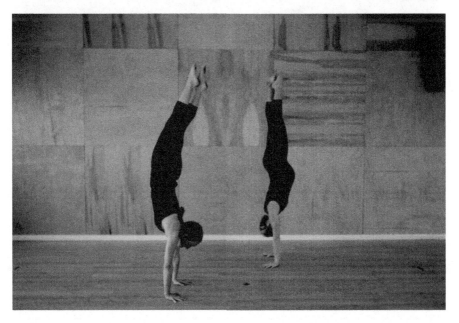

■◄ Once you feel comfortable holding your body up, you can start kicking up into a handstand. I would try this against the wall first, but eventually, the only way you will learn to do a handstand is by doing it! Start with hands up over your head. Split your stance so that your dominant foot is forward. In one motion, bring your hands down to the ground (the closer to your front foot the better) and kick your legs up. Stay looking at the ground between your hands.

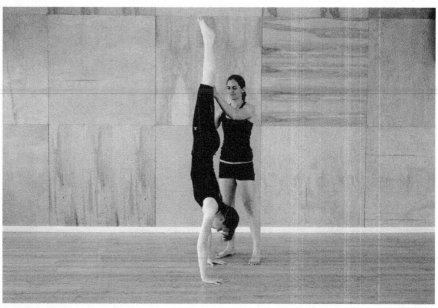

Bail out - You may have to practice this with a spotter first. You can also practice bailing out, by either rolling forward into a *tuck and roll*, or turning your hands so that you fall to the side smoothly.

ONE ARM PUSH-UP PROGRESSIONS

ONE ARM PUMP

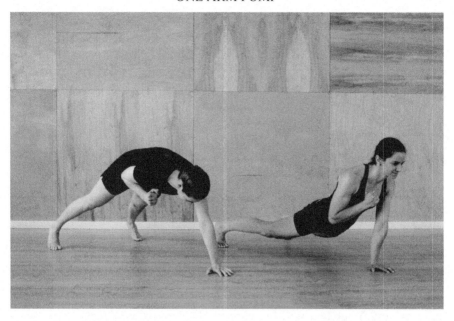

■◀ Start as for Push-Up Pump in the warm up. Do this with one hand instead.

ELEVATED HAND ON A BOX OR BENCH

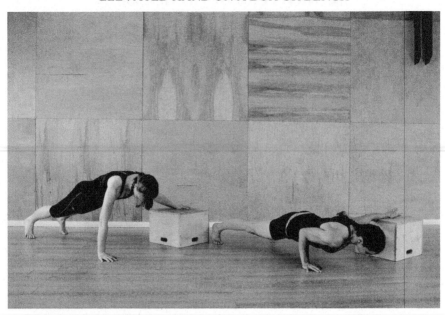

■◀ Start as for Push-Up, but bring one hand up to a box or bench to the side of you. Your feet will be wide in all one-arm variations. Keep your body tight as you lower down to the hand that is on the ground. Try to keep your body level to the ground.

ONE-ARM PUSH-UP

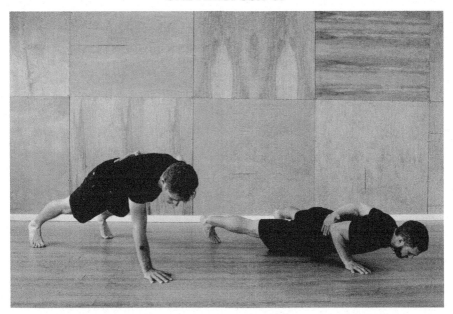

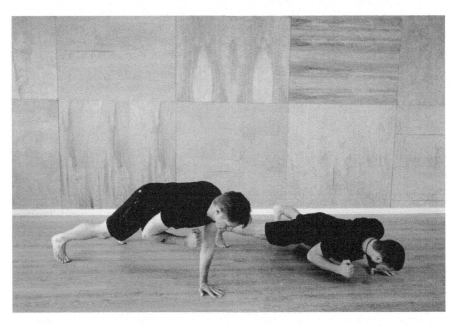

A legit one-arm push-up is done with the shoulders parallel to the floor, balls of the feet making contact with the floor, and lowering down until your chest almost touches the ground. Feet are slightly wider than shoulders. Fingers spread, weight on the heel of the palm. The hand should be placed just outside of the center. Point middle finger straight forward. The other hand can be placed on your lower back or on your thigh. Brace your body before lowering. Corkscrew and stomp through the heel of the palm to push back up.

ADVANCED TECHNIQUES

HANDSTAND PUSH-UP

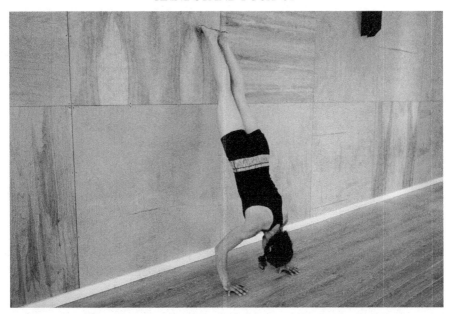

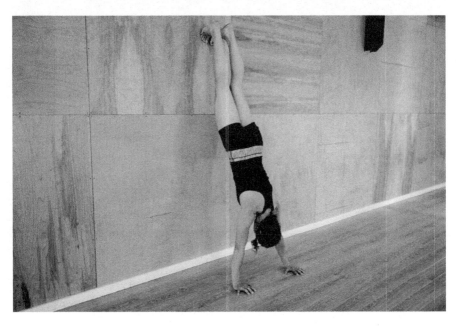

ONE ARM HINDU PUSH UP

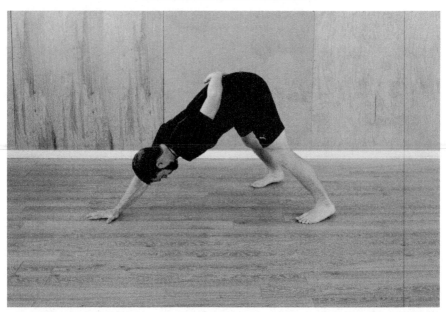

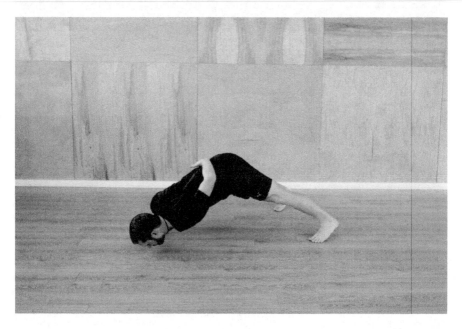

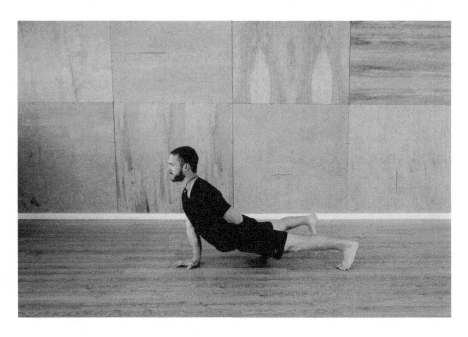

HINDU PUSH UP WITH HANDS STACKED

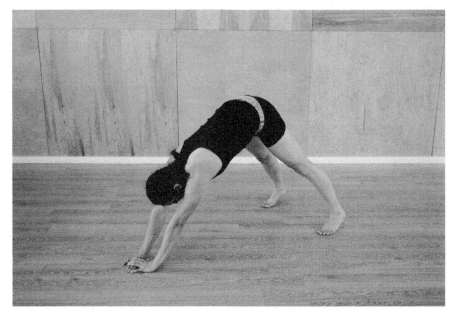

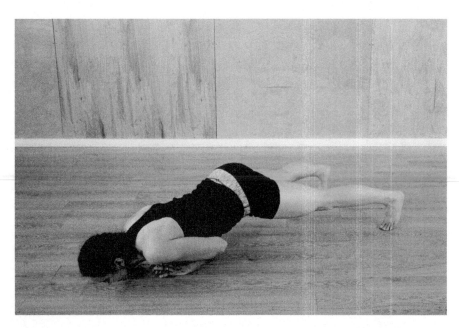

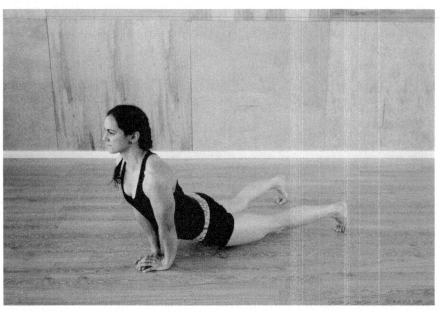

ONE ARM, ONE LEG PUSH UP

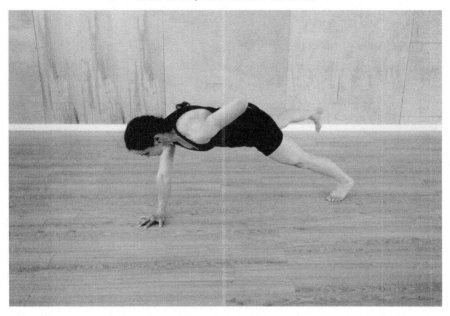

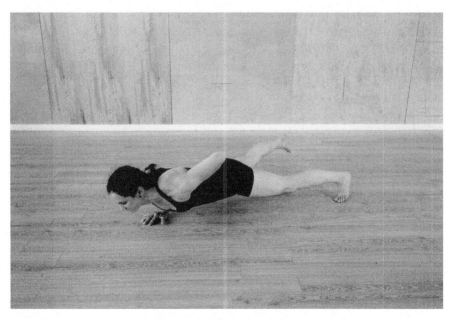

OTHER VARIATIONS

- Crow to Handstand
- One Arm Isometric Push Up
- One Arm Half Hindu Push Up
- One Leg, Two Arm Hindu Push Up

You can make any of the push-up variations harder or easier by changing the angle in which you do the push-up and points of contact. Make it harder by bringing the legs higher onto a box or the wall. Make them easier by bringing the hands higher onto a box or wall. Make them harder by changing the position of the hands or feet with either one hand off the ground or one foot off the ground. You can also add an unstable surface to your feet or hands to create a different type of challenge.

CONDITIONING

You can use any of the exercises listed above as a conditioning exercise. But for it to be a conditioning exercise, you must be able to complete high repetition of the movement (8+reps), so choose the exercises appropriately.

Here are a few conditioning push-up variations:
- Push-up with Leg Raise
- Push-up with Hand to Belly
- Push-up with Arm Raise
- Push-up with Leg Cross Through
- Spider Push-up
- Mountain Climbers

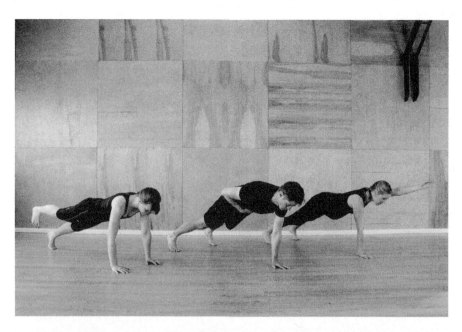

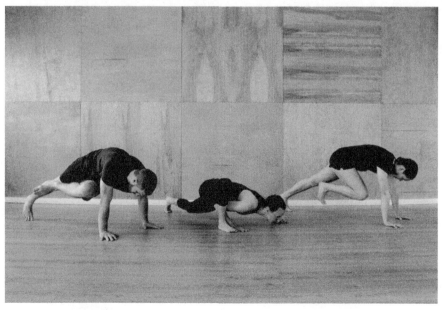

ADDING POWER

You can also make push-ups into a power exercise. The exercise selected needs to be easy enough to execute 1-3 reps. Some examples are:

- Clapping Push-Ups from the Ground 🎥
- Clapping Push-Ups from the Wall
- Push-Up to Kneeling 🎥

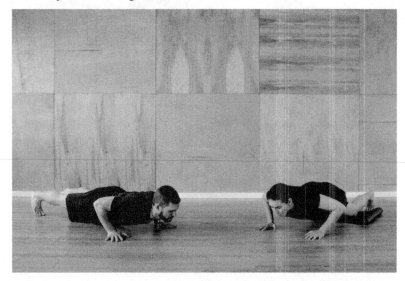

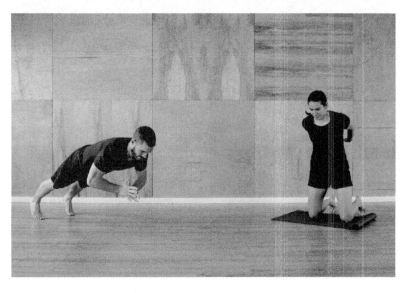

8

SECTION EIGHT

SQUAT VARIATIONS AND PROGRESSIONS

Basic Pistol Progression from the Testing Section

- Wall Squat
- Assisted 90-Degree Squat
- Squat to Box
- Assisted Full Squat
- Full Squat
- Feet Together Squat
- Single Leg Squat from Bench
- Pistol

Flip through the next few pages to see the variations of the Squat.

HINGE

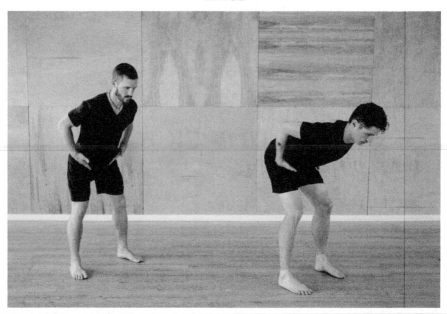

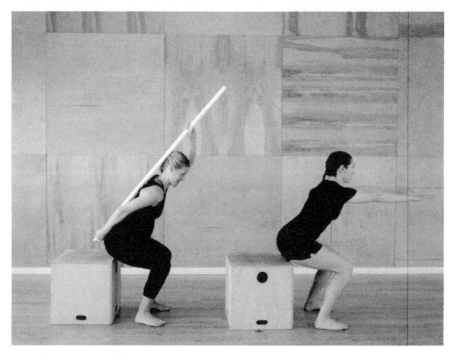

This is the most important movement to start with when beginning the squat progressions. Start with feet just wider than hips width apart. Put your pinkies on your hip creases. Push your pinkies back into the creases and allow this pressure to push your hips back. Bend your legs slightly as your hips come back. Then start again. You can also do this with a stick on your back, reinforcing good spinal position. Hold the stick along your spine. As you hinge, you are trying to maintain the contact points of your spine and head as you hinge. Don't let your knees bend just yet. Once you feel you have been able to execute this well, move onto the Squat to Box. Keep the stick on your spine and lower down, hinging first at the hips, then lower down to the box. Did you maintain contact with the stick?

ASSISTED 90-DEGREE SQUAT OR ASSISTED FULL SQUAT

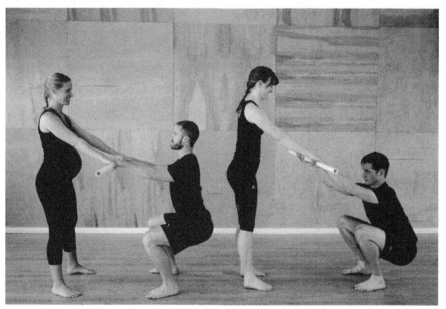

Start as for Full Squat. Hold a band or strap that is attached to something fixed. Focus on your weak points as you lower down. Go down as low as you can and hold as long as you can in the bottom position. Make corrections as you are down here, such as straightening out the spine, pushing your knees out, keeping sternum forward. Once you've had enough, return to standing.

90-DEGREE SQUAT OR BOX SQUAT

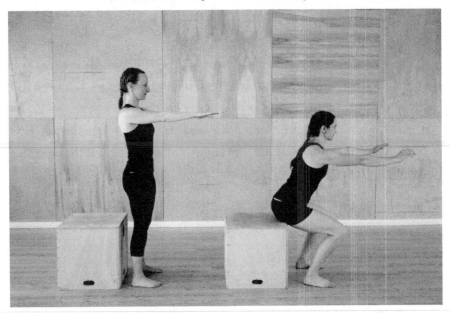

Start as for Full Squat, but go down to 90 degrees. Squeeze the glutes as much as you can before you ascend. To make this more challenging, you can hold the 90-degree position isometrically as long as you can.

FACE THE WALL SQUAT

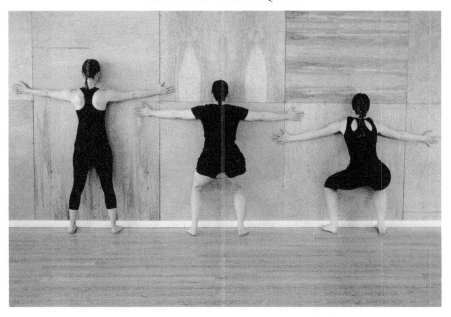

■◀ Start facing the wall and stand a few inches away from it. Mark this point. Then prepare as for 90-degree squat. Lower yourself down, trying not to touch the wall. This is a great exercise to teach you good spinal positioning and balance between your feet, hips and shoulders.

FULL SQUAT

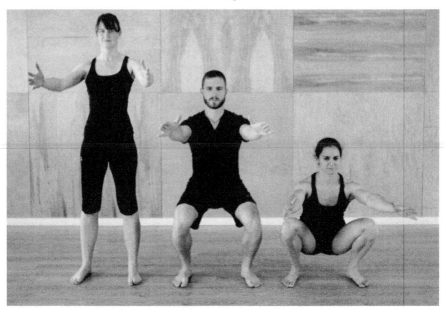

◼◀ Find a good stance with your feet. I usually like to take this stance just wider than my shoulders. Keep toes pointing straight forward. Stand with tension, abs and glutes tight with the head of the humerus rotated back into its socket. "Pull" yourself down, trying to keep your chest up and keeping your neck neutral inline with the spine. Knees should push out to the side. Don't let your knees fall in! (You may notice your feet naturally turning out at the bottom. Let your feet do what they need to, but don't let the arches fall in and keep the heels on the ground. Ideally, you want your toes to stay slightly forward during the movement). Go down as far as you can, keeping heels pushing through the ground, spine straight. Hold as long as you can at the bottom position. Make corrections while you are down here. Before ascending, squeeze the glutes to push you up to starting position.

FEET TOGETHER FULL SQUAT

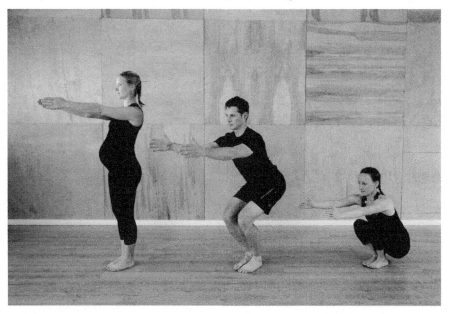

◼ This exercise helps increase flexibility for the Pistol. Start with feet together. Arms straight out in front. Lower yourself down as for Full Squat.

ROLL TO FULL SQUAT

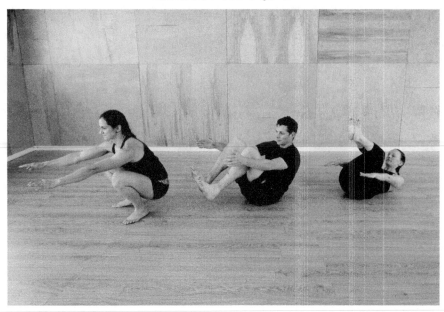

■◀ Start as for Full Squat. Squat all the way down. At the bottom, drop backwards and roll onto your back, then roll forwards so that you are in the bottom of Full Squat position again. The hard part is trying to get your butt up off the ground when you roll forward.

SISSY SQUAT

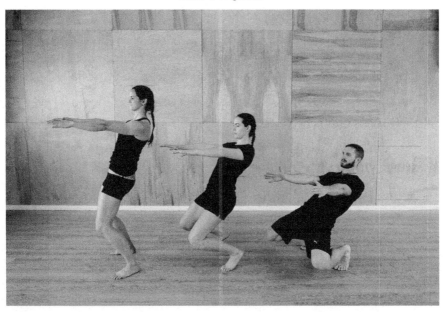

◀ This one is quite different to the other squat variations and is a great lead up to the Back Bend. Start standing straight, with tension! Keep your hips straight for this one. You will be hinging from the knees. Bend your knees down toward the ground. Your heels will come up off the ground and you will have to bend or lean back with arms out in front to counter weight your lower body. Go down as far as you can with control, then come back up.

ONE LEG PROGRESSIONS

LUNGES

Keeping your torso tight and knees inline with hips and ankles, take a step forward slowly. It should be far enough to have both knees at 90 degrees when you lower down. Lower down so that each knee comes to 90 degrees. The front shin should be vertical. Your weight should be evenly distributed between the front and back leg. Keep chest up. Step back into standing and switch legs. You can do this as an isometric exercise, holding the bottom position, or rep it out.

REVERSE LUNGES

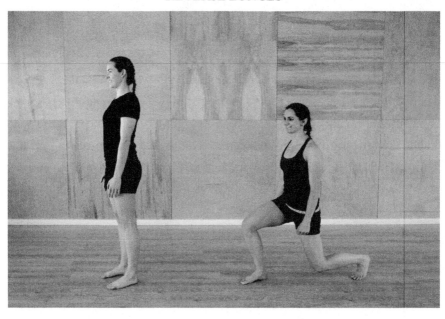

Same as for Lunges, but step backward. This variation is better for the knees if you have some patella issues.

ONE LEG ROMANIAN DEAD LIFT

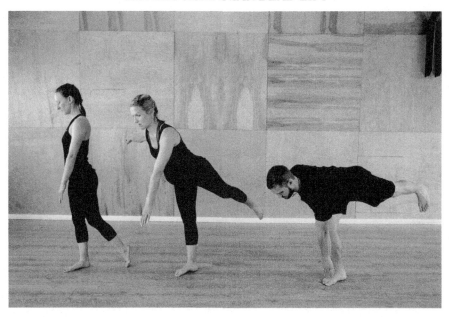

Start standing. Increase tension. The hand and leg of the same side of your body should move together. Bring the hand down toward the opposite foot and keep the leg straight. The back leg should drive up toward the ceiling. A straight line should be made from your heel to the shoulder. Keep hips straight, parallel to the ground. Come back up to the start.

BOX PISTOL

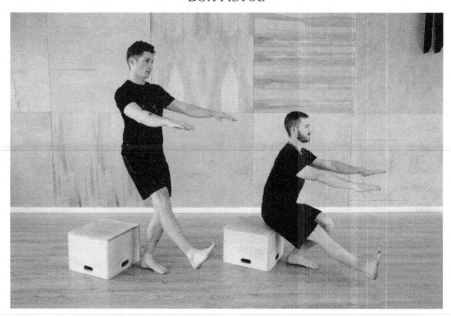

◼◣ Start as for Pistol. Keep shins as vertical as you can, you may need to drive the knee forward to leverage better, but do your best. Keeping the chin as vertical as you can places less stress on the patella tendon and increases tension in the hamstrings. Rock back on the box at the bottom; don't lose tension. Stand back up, "stomp" through the ground.

PISTOL

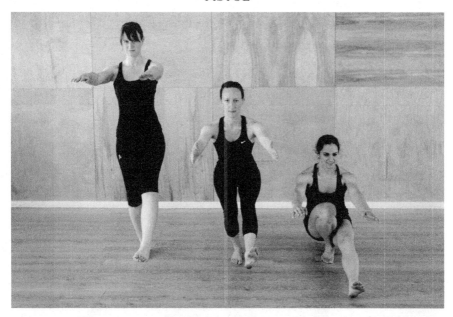

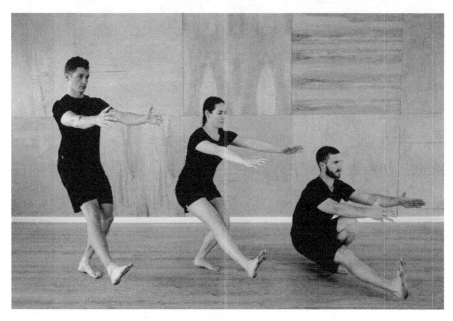

■◄ One leg comes forward out in front; keep it straight. Keep standing with shins vertical. Pretend you have a ski boot on. Hinge at the hips so that your butt comes back. Arms out in front. Don't lose tension at the bottom. Grip the floor with your toes. Inhale on the way down; exhale as you are about to lift up. Some folks may need to hold a counterweight to do a full pistol because of structure and build of the body. Important! Don't let your knee or ankle drop in, or let your body twist.

ROCKING PISTOL

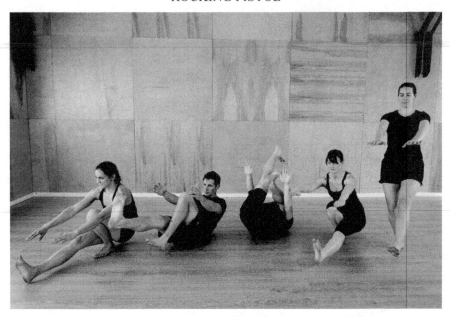

■◖ Start as for Pistol, go all the way down. At the bottom, rock onto your back, then rock forward into the bottom position of the pistol, and stand up.

HOLDING THE TOE PISTOL

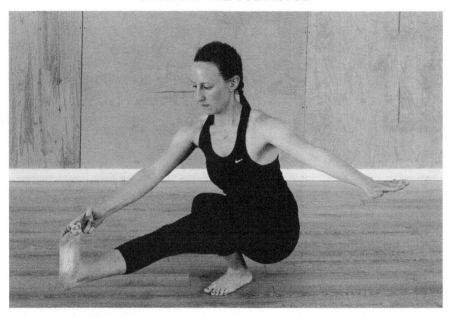

Same as for Pistol, but hold the toe with your hand in front of you. Try to keep your leg straight.

AIRBORNE LUNGE

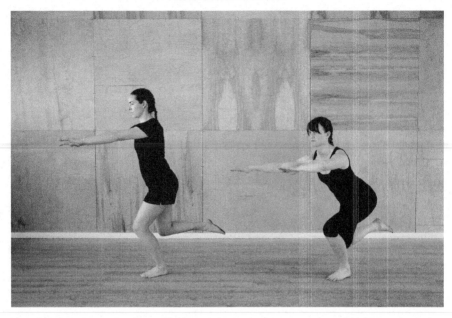

▶️ Start as for Pistol, but the back leg hovers off the ground behind you as you lower down. Lower down until the back knee lightly touches the ground. Return to start.

SHRIMP SQUAT

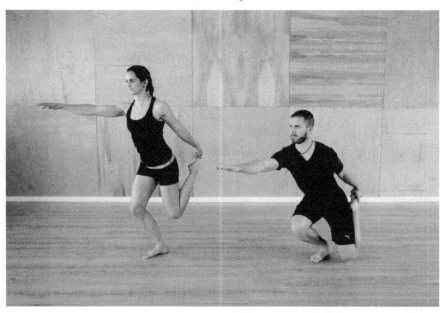

Start as for Pistol, but instead bend your knee and hold your foot behind you. Lower down until your knee lightly touches the ground and then come back up. As an alternative, you can use a box to tap the knee on to, but be careful not to bang your knee!

ADVANCED TECHNIQUES

SWITCH FEET

Go into a full squat. Slowly bring one leg out from under you without using your hands, and balance. Try to stand up from here. Another version is to do one pistol and at the bottom switch feet without losing balance, then stand up.

ONE LEG SQUAT OFF OF A BOX

Start on top of a box. Bring one leg off to the side, and squat down with the other leg. Go down as far as you can, then stand up.

ONE LEG SIDE AIRBORNE LUNGE

Just like the Airborne Lunge, but instead, the trailing leg is out to the side, off the ground. Try to keep that leg as straight as possible as you lower down.

CONDITIONING AND POWER

You can use any of the exercises listed above for conditioning purposes. But for it to be a conditioning exercise, you must be able to complete high repetition of the movement (8+reps). For it to be a power exercise, you must have very, very good technique and do fewer reps so you can focus on the execution (1-3reps); so choose the exercises appropriately. Listed below would be the progression for low intensity power to high intensity power:

- Side Lunges
- One Leg Box Step Up
- Speed Squats
- Speed Lunges
- Jump Squats
- Jumping Lunges
- Box Jumps
- One Leg Box Jumps

- Two Legged Bounding
- One Legged Bounding
- Depth Jumps

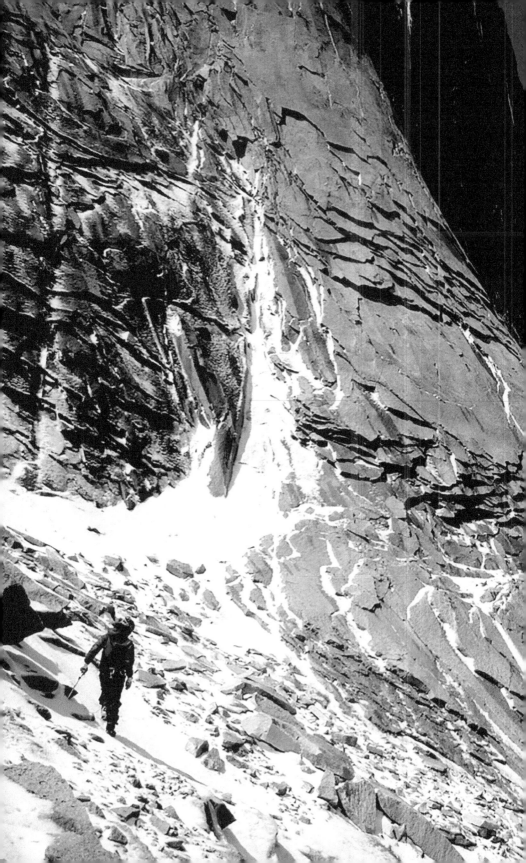

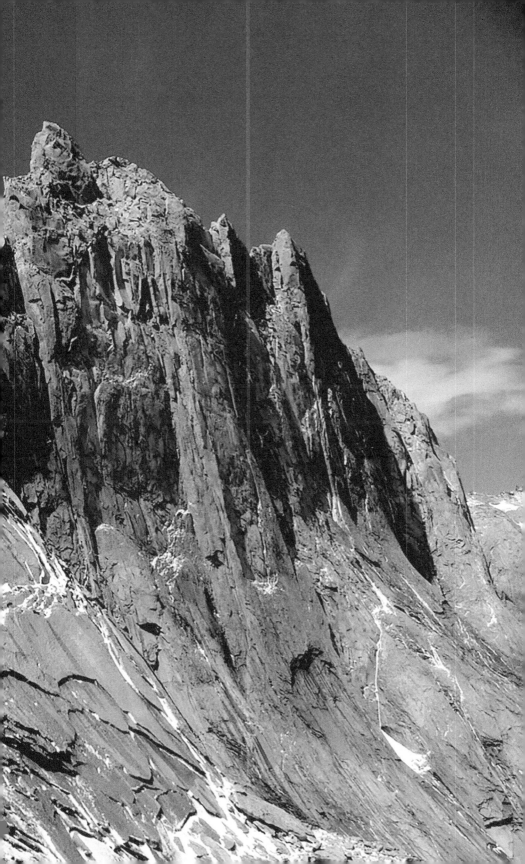

9

SECTION NINE

BACK BEND VARIATIONS AND PROGRESSIONS

Basic Back Bend Progression from the Testing Section

- Superman
- Bridge
- See-Saw
- From the ground back bend
- Camel
- Walk Hands down the Wall
- Back Bend

Flip through the next few pages to see the variations for the Back Bend.

SUPERMAN

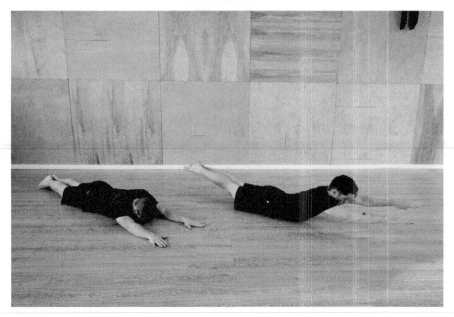

■◀ Start lying on the ground; face down. Arms extended overhead and big toes touching. Keep your neck neutral. Raise your arms and legs up off the ground. Keep arms and legs straight, holding tension!

HIP BRIDGE

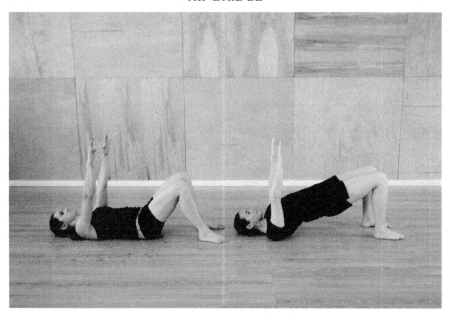

◼◀ Start on your back. Bend knees up so that your heels are fairly close to your hips, and hips width apart. Arms up in the air, hands inline with your shoulders. Press your back into the ground. Keep this tension then press your hips up to the ceiling as far as you can and hold.

COBRA

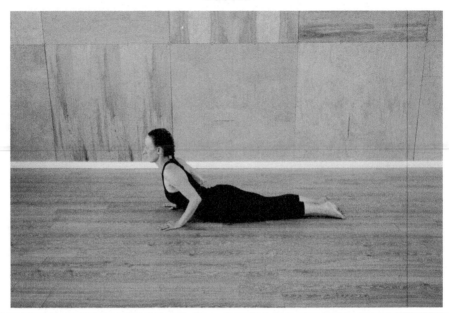

■◀ Start lying on the ground face down. Hands under your shoulders. Keep toes together and pointed. Slowly press your chest up off the ground. You can look up to the ceiling. Hold here.

SINGLE LEG BRIDGE

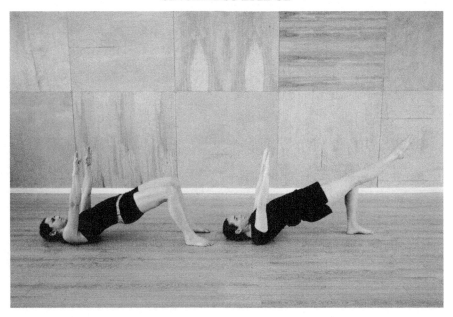

🎥 Start as for Hip Bridge. At the top, keep the tension and extend one leg. Try to keep the hips level.

STRAIGHT LEG BRIDGE

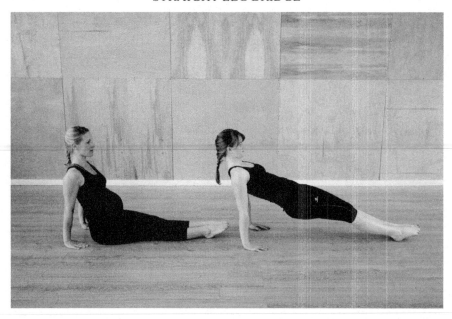

■ Start sitting on the ground. Legs extended out in front, heels and toes together, point your toes. Hands back behind the hips, fingers pointing toward the toes. Brace your torso, push your hips up. Keep chin tucked.

STRAIGHT SINGLE LEG BRIDGE

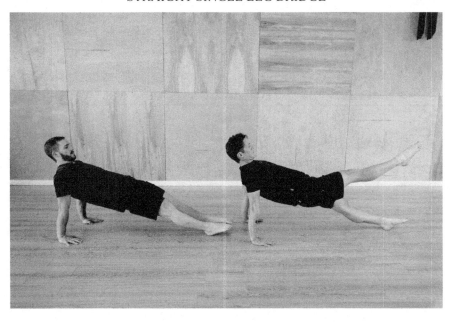

■◀ Start as for Straight Leg Bridge. Do this with one leg instead.

SINGLE ARM STRAIGHT LEG BRIDGE

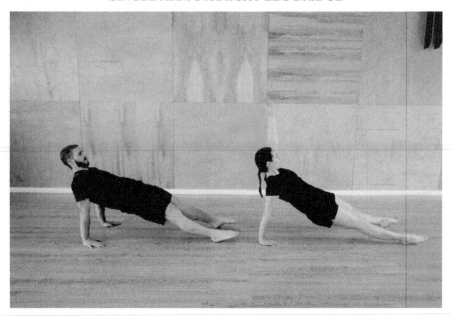

Start as for Straight Leg Bridge. Do this with one arm.

TABLE TOP

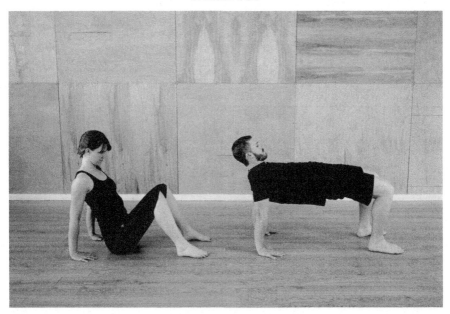

■◀ Start sitting with knees bent, feet close to the hips and hips width apart. Hands just behind the shoulders. Fingers can point forward or backward. Push hips up so that you are on your hands and your feet. Push through your heels of both your feet and hands.

TABLE TOP SINGLE LEG

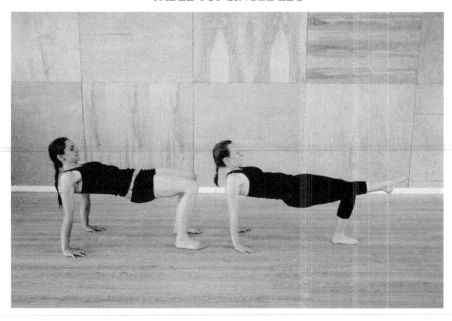

Start as for Table Top. At the top, extend one leg. You can also start the movement with just one leg. Keep hips straight.

TABLE TOP SINGLE ARM

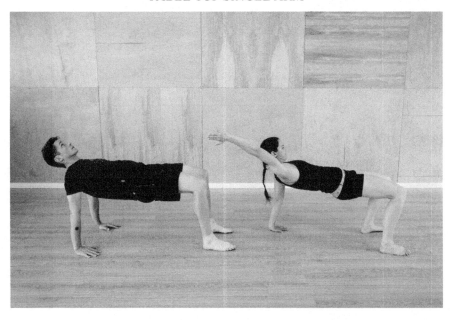

Start as for Table Top. At the top, raise one arm. You can also start the movement with one arm. Keep hips straight.

SCORPION MOVE

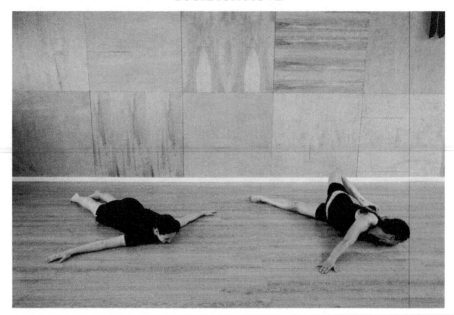

▶ Start lying on your belly. Hands stretched out to the side. Bring your right toe to the left hand, crossing your leg over the top of your body, feeling the stretch in your hip flexors. Bring the leg back down and switch legs. Try to look at the hand that you are bringing the toe to.

SEE-SAW

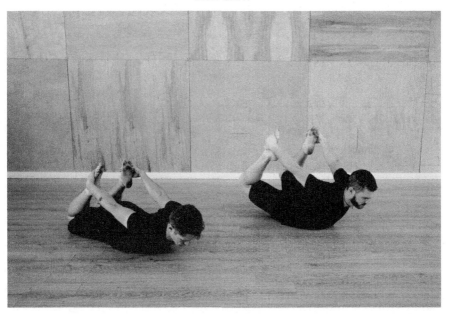

Start on your belly. Bring the feet into the hands behind you. Keep neck neutral. Push your feet up to the ceiling, which will bring your knees and shoulders up off the ground. Breathe here. Try to hold as long as you can. Keep neck neutral.

TOP OF HEAD BACK BEND

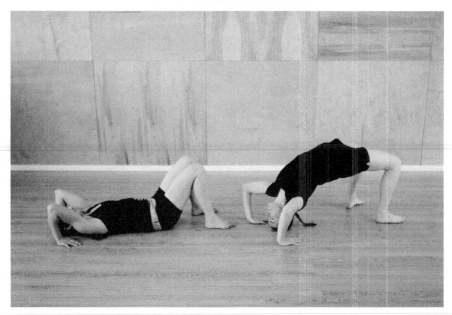

■◀ Start on your back. Bend knees, feet on the ground. Bring hands over the top of your shoulders and onto the ground. Elbows should point back behind you. Slowly push up and place the top of your head on the ground. Make sure that weight is evenly distributed on your feet, head and hands. Press hips up and extend a little farther.

FROM THE GROUND BACK BEND

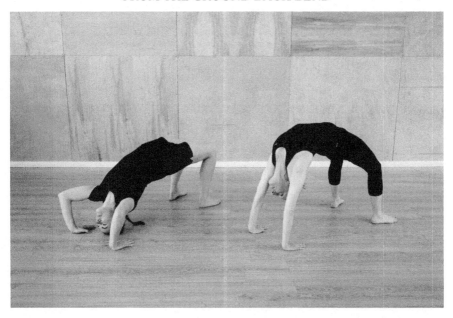

Start as for previous. Push all the way up to back bend. Try to keep weight evenly distributed. You are trying to look behind you, or towards your fingers.

CAMEL

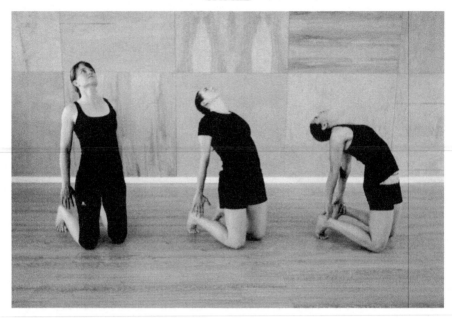

◼️ Start kneeling on the ground, knees hips width apart, toes tucked under. Pull your thighs inward. Hands on your sacrum. Keep chin tucked. Create tension in your torso. Inhale and lift your spine and press through the ground. Extend into a back bend. Press the hips forward and reach back to find your heels with palms facing out. Keep pressing hips forward, drop your head back and lift the chest up toward the ceiling. You can also try this with toes untucked.

WALK DOWN THE WALL BACK BEND

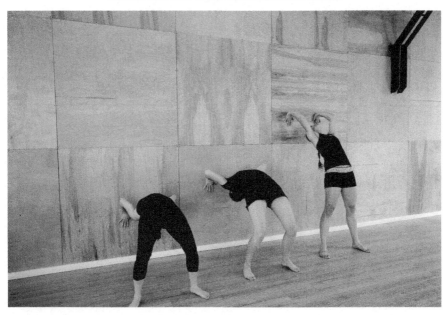

Stand a few feet from the wall, facing away. Use the same starting cues as for Back Bend. Reach back until you touch the wall. Slowly walk your hands down. Keep pushing your hips forward as you walk your hands down. Go down as far as you can.

BACK BEND

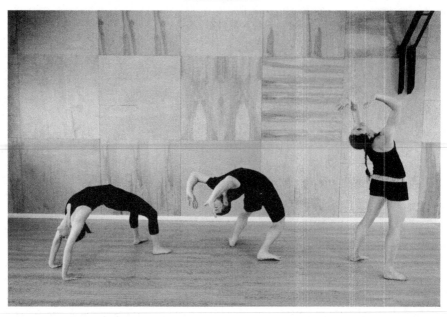

Feet should start wider than your hips. Tense up from the ground, pressing your heels into the ground, and follow tension up through your body. Your thighs should be engaged, "zipping up" your kneecaps (Kneecaps draw upward). Try to force some separation between your thighs without moving the feet. Lead with the arms going back, fingers pointing back. Keep abs slightly tense. Look back at your hands, and try to find the ground. Keep leading with your eyes to the ground. Don't let your glutes squeeze too much, instead try to tilt the pubic bone upward. Reach back slowly until your hands make contact with the ground. Press your heels into the ground. Try to relax your breath and keep it constant.

ADVANCED TECHNIQUES

A fun advanced variation of the back bend is the Back Bend Walk Over, which can be done with a partner if you have never attempted it before. Make sure that you can do a back bend from the ground, as well as feel confident in the handstand before attempting this one.

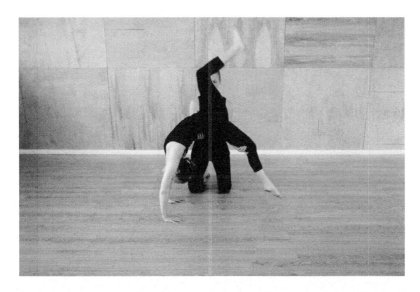

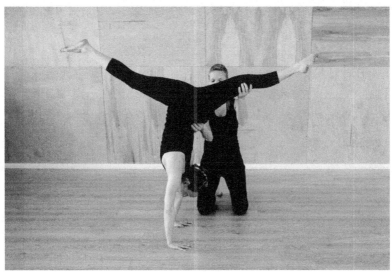

Now that you have seen numerous variations, and maybe you have tried some of these as you read through them, it's time to apply these movements to your practice and training. But first, you have to choose your target exercise.

SECTION TEN

PROGRAMS AND PRACTICE

Now it's time to put movement into practice. First choose a goal for movement. What is it that you want to achieve? Where do you have weaknesses? Maybe you want to do a one-leg pistol and be able to do a push-up with a totally straight body. Then those need to be your focus. Practice two goals each day and work on their variations.

Don't forget to download your free programs based on the book! Download them at www.SimpleStrengthBook.com

TARGET EXERCISE

I've chosen two exercises from each movement and given you an example of which test to do and what exercises to work up to in order to get to your target movement. First you must test your body to see if you have the range of motion to execute the target movement. You also want to check for any aches and pains associated with the test movement first before doing the target movement.

In order to get better at your target movements you need to spend time doing them. In the following pages, I will show you a test and then the progressions for each.

You can use the following as a template for your training or practice sessions. I suggest practicing each target movement for 2-5 minutes.

Follow those up with strength/progression exercises. Choose 2-3 exercises from the lists. Complete 8-10 reps of each movement, rest 1-2 minutes between each exercise. Repeat for up to 3-5 sets. Remember, you want to end fresh, not completely worn out from all of the work.

Pistol

Test: Full Bodyweight Squat holding 3-4 minutes.

You are clear to work on Pistols if you have no pain in the joints and you can execute the squat with good technique.

Progression: Try the Pistol first. Spend a few minutes every other day working on it. To build strength for this exercise, you can incorporate the single leg squat to a box. If you can execute the single leg to the box, you can move onto the air lunge and shrimp squat. But if Pistols are your target, you need to work on Pistols!

Full Squat

Test: 90-degree squat or assisted full squat.

If you can perform a squat to 90-degrees at your knee joint without compensating with your feet or knees, then you can move on to a full squat. If your heels start coming up, or if you feel tightness, use an assist to help you further down into the motion.

Progression: If your target is a full squat, then this is where you need to spend a lot of your time. The full squat is more of a mobility exercise than a strength exercise if you can already execute the 90-degree squat. You need to teach your body to open up in the bottom position of the full squat. Work up to 10 minutes in the full squat with or without an assist.

Handstand

Test: A-Frame push-up

The thing about handstands is that if you haven't done it since you were a kid, you may have lost some proprioception to being inverted, and also the ability to hold your body up with your arms. The best place to start is the A-Frame Push-Up.

Progression: The A-Frame Push-Up is a great way to know if you can handle at least half your bodyweight. If you can execute around 5-10 reps of great A-Frame push-ups, then move onto the Face the Wall Handstand. The aim here is to get you used to being upside down and to build strength for the handstand. But, the only way you will get better at handstands is to do handstands. So, test first, using a spotter if needed, then if you are comfortable, spend five minutes every other day working on handstands and then practice strength exercises after.

Push-Up
Test: Plank + Bench Push-Up
If you can keep good form and tension in your core during 10-20 Bench Push-Ups, you are ready to tackle the full Push-Up. Practicing the Plank position is crucial to get into the initial set up of Push-Up, as well as making sure there are no aches and pains.
Progression: Practice the Push-Up, with the best form as possible for two minutes every other day. Work on Not the Knee Push Up, A-Frame Holds, and Cobra as strength exercises.

Back Bend
Test: Back Bend from the Floor + Camel
Having the flexibility to execute Back Bends from the Floor, plus the strength of going into Camel and holding Camel for a few minutes will be a good indicator to move onto back bends.
Progression: If you can't do the back bends yet from standing, the best way to work up to it is to practice walking the hands down the wall. Practice this a few minutes every other day. Work on Backward Spinal Bends, Sissy Squats, and holding Camel as strength and mobility exercises after your Back Bend practice.

Camel

Test: See Saw + Top of Head Back Bend

This move is about opening up the chest, and having the ability to breathe while in this position. The Top of the Head Back Bend can give you great feedback on how your body reacts to being inverted, and if your breath can continue in this position. If you can hold this for a few minutes, you can move onto Camel. Your knees might also play a part in this move, so make sure you can kneel down and put pressure on your kneecaps.

Progression: Superman and Backward Spinal Bends for strength and mobility.

Below are three basic progression programs for a PRACTICE ORIENTED program. Start with two minutes of practice with the intention of working up to five minutes. For the strength component of practice, I have included times to work on it. I prefer this to specifying a number of repetitions because it keeps my attention and focus up and doesn't bring me to failure. If you can only complete three repetitions of the best movement possible, so be it. Each week, you can add 20-30 seconds to each set, or add another set to the exercise.

To make the programs more challenging each week, you can either add one minute to the conditioning portion of the workouts or go around the conditioning portion of the workout as a circuit and add a circuit round each week.

BEGINNER PROGRAM

	Day 1 Activity	Time (min)	Day 2 Activity	Time (min)	Day 3 Activity	Time (min)	Day 4 Activity	Time (min)	Day 5 Activity	Time (min)	Day 6 Activity	Day 7 Activity
Daily Practice Goals	Target	4	Target	4	Target	4	Target	4	Target	4	Big Day Outside	Big Day Outside
	Focused Strength	6			Focused Strength	4			Focused Strength	6		
	Conditioning	3			Conditioning	8			Conditioning	3		
Warm Up	Warm Up	4	Warm Up	4	Warm Up	4	Warm Up	4	Warm Up	4		
Target	Push up	2	Full Squat	4	A-Frame Push up	2	Full Squat	4	Push Up	2		
	Camel	2			Camel	2			Camel	2		
Focused Strength	Plank	2			Push up With Leg Raise alt with Arm Raise	2			Plank	2		
	A-Frame Hold	2			Superman	2			Superman	2		
	Spinal back bends	2							Spinal back bends	2		
Conditioning	Bench Push Ups	1			Jumping Jacks	2			Bench Push Ups	1		
	Jump squats from Box	1			Squat to box	2			Jump squats From box	1		
	Walking Lunges	1			Face the Wall Squats	2			Walking Lunges	1		
					Beast Crawl	2						
Total Time (mins)	17		8		20		8		17			

SIMPLE STRENGTH · 165

INTERMEDIATE PROGRAM

	Day 1 Activity	Day 1 Time (min)	Day 2 Activity	Day 2 Time (min)	Day 3 Activity	Day 3 Time (min)	Day 4 Activity	Day 4 Time (min)	Day 5 Activity	Day 5 Time (min)	Day 6 Activity	Day 7 Activity
Daily Practice Goals	Target	4	Target	4	Target	4	Target	4	Target	4		
	Focused Strength	6			Focused Strength	4			Focused Strength	6		
	Conditioning	3			Conditioning	8			Conditioning	3		
Warm Up	Warm Up	4	Warm Up	4	Warm Up	4	Warm Up	4	Warm Up	4		
Target	Handstand	2	Pistol	4	One Arm PU	2	Handstand	4	Camel	2		
	Camel	2	Squat		Camel	2			Pistol	2		
Focused Strength	A-Frame Push up	2			Hindu Push up	2			A-Frame Push up	2	Big Day Outside	Big Day Outside
	Face to Wall Holds	2			Single Leg Squat to Box	2			Face the Wall Holds	2		
	Spinal back Bends	2							Spinal back bends	2		
Conditioning	Push ups	1			Jumping Lunges	2			Push ups	1		
	Jump Squats	1			Full Squat	2			Jump Squats	1		
	Speed Squats	1			Beast Crawl	2			Speed Squats	1		
					Superman	2						
Total Time (mins)	17		8		20		8		17			

ADVANCED PROGRAM

	Day 1		Day 2		Day 3		Day 4		Day 5		Day 6	Day 7
	Activity	Time (min)	Activity	Time (min)	Activity	Time (min)	Activity	Time (min)	Activity	Time (min)	Activity	Activity
Daily Practice Goals	Target	4	Target	4	Target	2	Target	4	Target	4		
	Focused Strength	6			Focused Strength	6			Focused Strength	6		
	Conditioning	4			Conditioning	8			Conditioning	3		
Warm Up	Warm Up	4	Warm Up	4	Warm Up	4	Warm Up	4	Warm Up	4		
Target	Handstand Push Up	2	Isometric Pistols	4	One Arm PU	2	Handstand	4	Back Bend	2		
	Back Bend	2					Isometric Pistol	4	One Arm Push Up	2		
Focused Strength	Face the wall Push Up	2			Switch Feet Pistol	2			A-Frame Push Up	2	Big Day outside	Big Day Outside
	Back Bend from the Ground	2			Fin Push Ups	2			Face the Wall Holds	2		
	Spinal back Bends	2			Shrimp Squat	2			Scorpions	2		
Conditioning	Push ups	1			Hindu Push ups	2			Jumping Lunges	1		
	Jump Squats	1			Jump Squats	2			Box Jumps	1		
	Clapping Push Ups	1			Spider Crawl	2			Beast Crawl	1		
	360 Jumps	1			Speed Squats	2						
Total Time (mins)	18		8		20		12		17			

SECTION ELEVEN

MOBILITY AND INCREASING
JOINT RANGE OF MOTION

THE DIFFERENCE BETWEEN
FLEXIBILITY AND MOBILITY

Flexibility implies that stretching will fix the problem, but really, mobility would be more accurate, as you need to fix many other issues than just "short muscles." The word *flexibility* means that the tissues and joints are passively stretched *without load*. When you put joints, tissues and fascia under load, it wouldn't be considered flexibility. This is why professionals use *mobility* as the term to describe most degrees of motion, as well as describing many movement issues. According to Gray Cook, the word *mobility* encompasses the anatomical definition to demonstrate joint mobility and soft tissue extensibility.

Ligaments and tendons are made of collagen and elastin. Collagen gives ligaments and tendons strength, and elastin provides them with elasticity. As you age, the elastin:collagen ratio changes in favor of collagen, or scar tissue. Exercise builds up micro trauma in your muscles, tendons and fascia, and when it heals, it forms scar tissue. The more that scar tissue lays down and less movement that happens in the tissues usually result in mobility problems. Gil Hedley has a great YouTube video (https://youtu.be/_FtSP-tkSug) showing how scar tissue, or "fuzz" is laid down if you don't move around enough or regularly. Gil is a riot; you have to see this video. Warning: it shows examples through the use of human cadavers.

THE NERVOUS SYSTEM

Your nervous system and how it relates to your fascia plays a big part in how *flexible* and *mobile* you are. Previously I talked about fascia as being a web that connects all tissue in the body together. Usually it is how the nervous system is communicating with the fascia during your movement, and where tight spots lie, that dictate your full range of motion. Tight spots happen because you either use one part of the joint too much, or the other part of the joint too little, causing an imbalance of tension. If there is *imbalance* of tension between the muscles surrounding the joints, which, with the laws of physics and fascia, this will affect the tension in other parts of your body. Being inflexible doesn't mean that you have 'short' muscles, it just means that the nervous system isn't used to letting your muscles slide out to full length, and possibly using tension in one area incorrectly to protect itself. This explanation is a little esoteric, but I think it is pertinent to understand flexibility correctly, rather than just thinking that if you stretch, your muscles will lengthen.

MOBILITY EXERCISES

There are some mobility techniques out there that are beyond the scope of this book, but I will share with you one technique that uses tension to strengthen the muscles as they lengthen, as well as teach the nervous system that it will be okay to go beyond certain points of extension. Normally, your body won't allow a new range of motion that it cannot control.

All of these exercises require you to hold tension as long as you can stand it. For the lower body exercises, you can usually go all out, but for the upper body exercises, pay particular attention to the shoulder joints, making sure not to *overstretch* the joint.

Flip through the next few pages to see the Mobility exercises.

FULL SQUAT STRETCH

Start in a full squat. You can use an assist if your heels are coming off the ground, or if you can't stay balanced. If you are using an assist, just focus on this position, and try to relax and move around in this bottom position. If you can stay in the full squat with no assist, you can do these following variations to increase your hip mobility and spinal strength. With each position, hold it for a few seconds with tension, and then come back out of tension. The goal is to accumulate around 10 seconds of tension, and repeat 3-5 times.

Variation #1: Twist

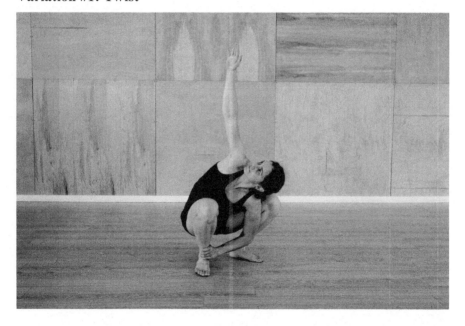

Variation #2: With Bar

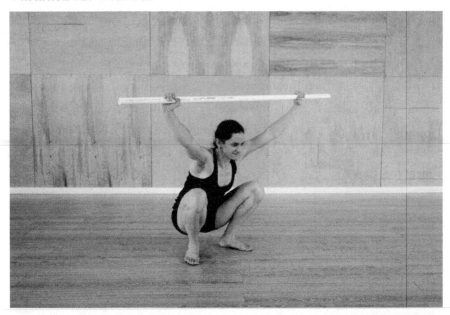

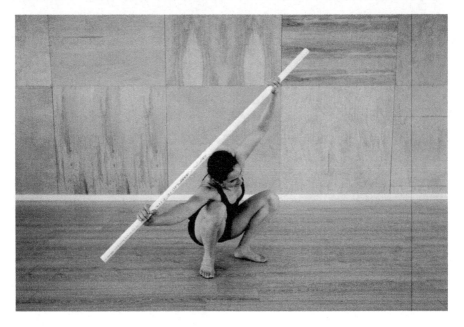

Variation #3: Hands at Prayer

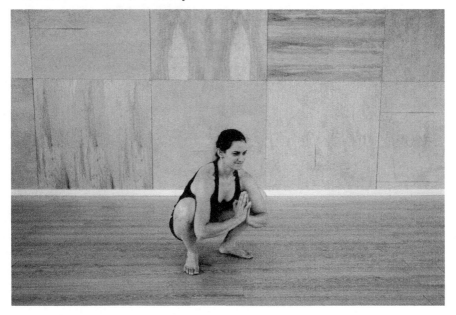

LUNGE AND TWIST

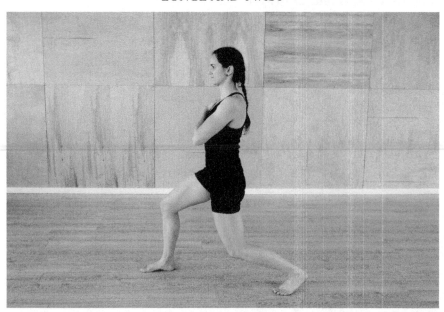

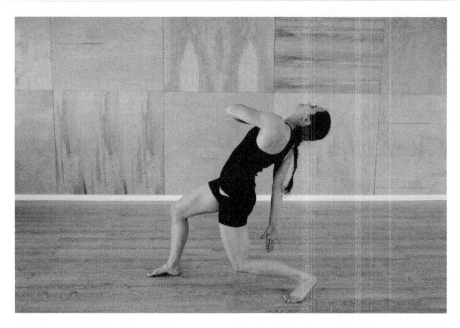

■ Start as for the Reverse Lunge position. Start with the right foot back. Place your right hand on your left shoulder. The goal is to reach your left hand to your right ankle. Don't try to twist from the hips, rather, extend throughout the spine and twist from the thorax and waist. You should feel an intense hip flexor stretch. You will also notice your obliques and muscles around the ribs working to keep you in a twisted position. This is great for balance too. Hold this twist for a few seconds with tension, or as long as you can stand it, breathe, and then come back out of tension. The goal is to accumulate around 10 seconds of tension, and repeat 3-5 times on each side.

BICEPS AND SHOULDERS

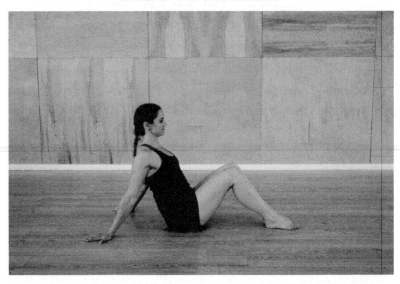

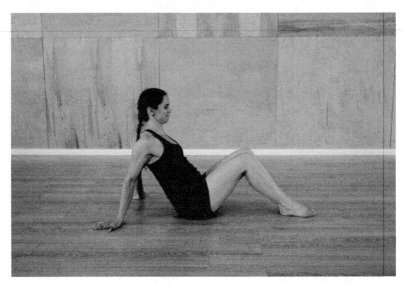

◼◣ Sit on the floor with your knees bent and your arms behind you, fingers pointing back. The arms should be slightly bent. The arms should come back until there is a slight stretch in the biceps and shoulders. Create tension in the arms by adding pressure to the palms and pulling the palms towards your hips, but without your hands moving. Hold the tension for a few seconds, breathe, and then come back out of tension. You may notice when you go back into tension, that you have gained some range of motion already. If this is you, take your hands back a bit more, or move your hips slightly forward. The goal is to accumulate around 10 seconds of tension, and repeat 3-5 times.

OVERHEAD REACH ELBOW PLANK

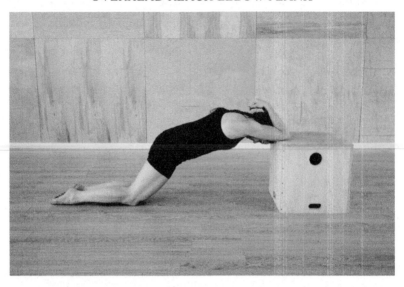

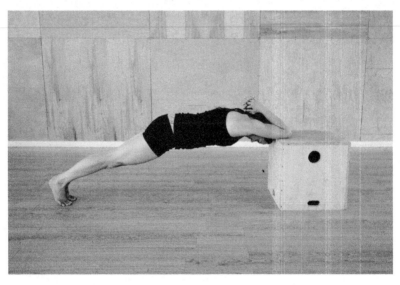

This one is for increasing thoracic range of motion. Go slowly with this progression because they can get very challenging. Make sure to have a mat for your knees and something high enough to place your elbows on, such as a bench or a box. Kneel down in front of a box and place your elbows on the edge of the box, and try to keep the hands close to the shoulders. Walk your knees back slowly, increasing the stretch in your armpit (there shouldn't be any pain; if there is, come out of it and try to reposition). In this position, add tension to your torso. Brace your core, keeping the abs flat. Breathe. If this is doable, try walking your knees even further back. And then finally, try the full plank position. Hold the position for a few seconds with tension, and then come back out of tension. The goal is to accumulate around 10 seconds of tension, and repeat 3-5 times.

STANDING HAMSTRING STRETCH

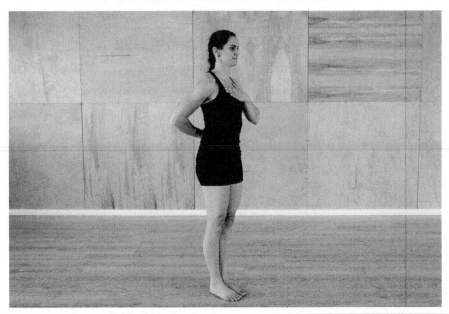

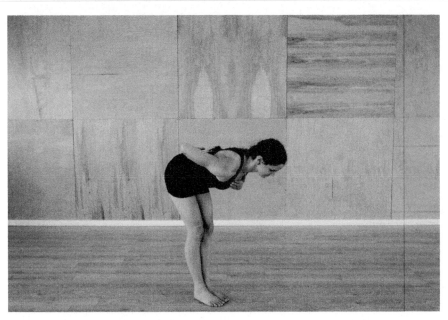

This is a variation of the straight-legged stretch, but you are adding tension from the beginning. Start standing with feet touching and knees locked out. Place a hand on your chest, and the other hand on your lower back. The hands are there to give you feedback on your spinal position. The goal for your spine is to stay straight. Hinge from the hips and lower your upper body down as far as you can while maintaining good spinal position. You should feel a great deal of stretch in the hamstrings and behind the knees. Breathe.

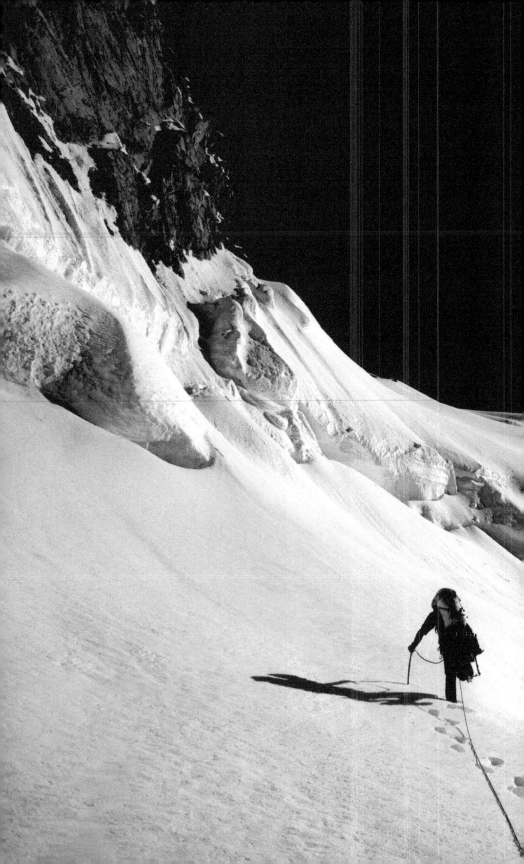

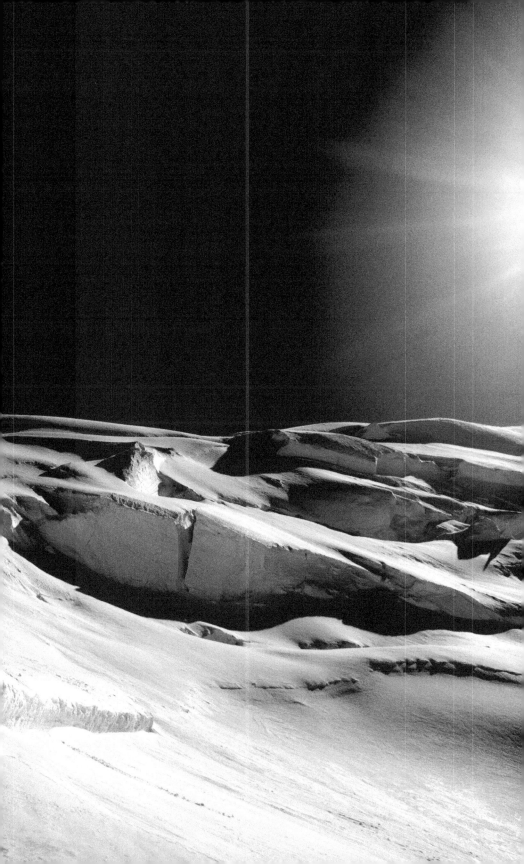

SECTION TWELVE

BEYOND BODYWEIGHT EXERCISE

Is Bodyweight Exercise Superior to Other Types of Resistance Training?

This is a tough question for me to give a short answer. It comes down to your goals. I think that for an outdoor athlete who has limited time and needs to recover fast, bodyweight exercise is a good option. You can also add in quick barbell workouts, such as cleans, dead lifts and snatches. These types of exercises are great for developing explosive strength; something that bodyweight exercise won't effectively deliver.

Changing it Up

I really enjoy doing different types of exercise. I practice handstands, pistols and back bends a few times a week. I also add in kettlebell practice and a ton of pulling exercises on the rings and on climbing holds. Sometimes I like to add in dead lifts to see how my strength is increasing. I have been able to increase my dead lift load without performing dead lifts. I have become stronger due to increased focus and tension during exercise.

Being Great Across a Variety of Skills

Some argue that doing several sports or several types of exercise won't make you great at any of them, just mediocre. I highly disagree. Movement patterns are inherently similar in athletics. If you can develop good body awareness and movement, you can recreate new patterns much faster. It wouldn't take long to become pretty decent at something new. And, if you love doing several different types of activities or sports, why hold yourself back? Practice the similar movements as much as you can and dedicate a few months to getting better technique in one area. Then, when you eventually come back, you will be able to do it 'off the couch'.

WRAPPING THINGS UP

Now that you have the knowledge to move forward with your program, I challenge you to stick with this program for four weeks. Refer to the Habits Section in Chapter 3 and use a calendar to cross off the days you complete a workout or practice, and start seeing your progress.

Be mindful in your days. Not just in movement, but in conversation, while you eat, how you sleep, how you treat your relationships. If you do this, you increase the quality of your life. Be your own project, make the most of it and enjoy.

All my best to you, and keep up the good work.

RECOMMENDED READING LIST

- *Essentials of Strength and Conditioning* by Thomas R. Baechle & Roger W. Earle
- Any book written by Pavel Tsatsouline
- *Movement* by Gray Cook
- *Oiling the Hinges* by Jarlo Ilano & Ryan Hurst
- *Anatomy Trains* by Thomas W. Myers

RECOMMENDED WEBSITES

- GMB Fitness - Smart Exercise for Physical Autonomy - http://gmb.io/
- Breaking Muscle - http://breakingmuscle.com/
- James Clear - http://jamesclear.com/
- MobilityWOD - http://www.mobilitywod.com/

A BIG THANK YOU

Thank you for purchasing this book and giving it a read. My goal is to continue improving the content in this book and will release new editions over time with updated information. You are welcome to contact me with questions or concerns at info@modusathletica.com. If you enjoyed reading it, please write a review on Amazon. You are also welcome to send this book to anyone of your friends and family.

I also wanted to say thank you to Aaron Rourke for the photos and Truc Allen for the videos. Thanks to my models Stephen, Katherine, Gwen, Brenda, Natalie, and Jake. Thank you to my partner in book crime Jonathan Cragle for keeping me on track. Thank you to all my clients, friends and supporters, you are all the reason why I do what I do!

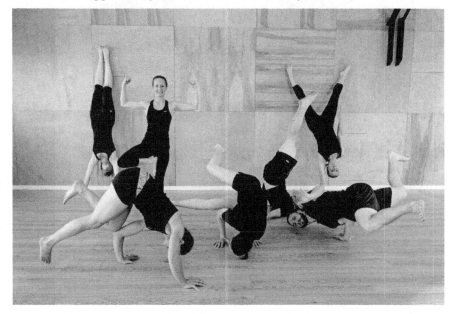

ABOUT THE AUTHOR

Mercedes Pollmeier is a Performance Coach based out of Seattle. She has a Master's degree in Human Movement and is committed to continuing her education in all fields related to training. She currently trains her athletes in person and online. If you'd like more information on her programs, what she offers, and free training articles, go to ModusAthletica.com.

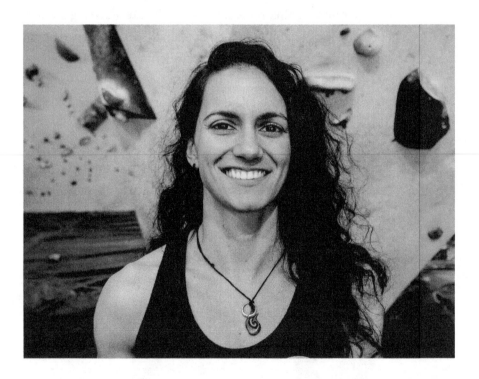

IMAGE CREDITS

After copyright page: Scott Bennett approaching the South Face of K6 in the Pakistani Karakoram during the summer of 2015. Photo credit: Graham Zimmerman.

After dedication page: Graham Zimmerman bouldering on the beautiful granite blocs around basecamp in the Nangmah Valley of the Pakistani Karakoram. Photo credit: Graham Zimmerman.

After table of contents: The stunning Changi Tower (6500m) above the Lechit Glacier in the Pakistani Karakoram, first ascended by Graham Zimmerman, Scott Bennett and Steve Swenson in the summer of 2015. Photo credit: Graham Zimmerman.

Page 2: Graham Zimmerman leading very enjoyable mixed climbing while making an attempt on a new route on the North face of Mt Dickey in Alaska during the spring of 2012. Photo credit: Joe Sambataro.

Page 5: Scott Bennett looks out at the Diamond on Long Peak Colorado. Photo credit Graham Zimmerman.

Page 65: Steve Swenson and Hajji Rasool walking out from basecamp in the Nangmah Valley of Pakistan. Photo credit: Graham Zimmerman.

Page 138: Ian Nicholson checking out climbing options during a brief spell of good weather in the French Valley of Torres Del Paine National Park in Chilean Patagonia during January 2010. Photo credit: Graham Zimmerman.

Page 182: Scott Bennett climbing the final snow and ice fields towards the summit of K6 West (7040m) while making the first ascent of the Southwest Ridge in 2015. Photo credit: Graham Zimmerman.

Made in the USA
Las Vegas, NV
29 December 2021